'Y? OGA

Shanti Troy Cox

(Meditator 20+ Years- Yoga Instructor 12+ Years)

The Y? of Yoga. Why is yoga popular?

There is so much Yoga and so many styles, how does one navigate the maze of options and find the right Yoga or teacher?

Avoid the pitfalls of modern Yoga through this guidebook with the help of an experienced teacher's insight and the stories of people like you who have found results in this Yoga expose.

"*Yoga is popular. What is popular is NOT Yoga.*"-Yogi Amrit Desai

Why do you do yoga?

"Yoga requires me to stay in the moment at all times." Claire N.

"The classes are spiritually restorative."- Loraine W.

"I like Troy's' classes 'true yoga' and not some calisthenics gym type work out. I love the practice of yoga as body, mind, and spirit. The body mind connecting practices allow the spirit to rise up."- Bob B.

"When you talk to Troy, you can see his passion for what he does. He wants to help guide you on your journey with yoga."- Elvira V.

"The warm and welcome atmosphere. Wide variety of lessons to choose from. Many thanks to Troy."- Jeny V.

"Troy is a true Yogi and an excellent instructor, No pretense here." Dina K.

"His technical cues are perfectly matched to the essence of each movement & the closing thoughts are beautifully spoken."- Donna

"Troy's classes are wonderful. I love that I can pick a restorative session or a more challenging one depending on how I'm feeling on a particular day to pursue my love of yoga!"- Allison B.

- First Name Ramdas

- State/Province Utah

- Country USA

- Age 30 - 44

- Type of Yoga do You practice? Amrit Yoga

- How long have you practiced Yoga? 13 years

  Why do/ did you practice Yoga?

Initially because it made me easier to be around for my family. With continued practice, I've gone from living a life of depression and suicidal thoughts and attempts to a life absolutely free of depression, one that is full of joy and peace. It also helps my creaky body feel pretty good too.

- First Name Michelle

- State/Province CA

- Country USA

- Age 30 - 44

- Type of Yoga do You practice? Hatha

- How long have you practiced Yoga? 2 years

  Why do/ did you practice Yoga?

I practice yoga for my health. Maintaining flexibility, quieting my mind and breathing techniques.

- First Name Lorie DeHimer
- State/Province VT
- Country USA
- Age 45 - 60
- Type of Yoga do You practice? Amrit--Hatha Bhakti, Giana
- How long have you practiced Yoga? 10 years

     Why do/ did you practice Yoga?

To learn how to be like a yogi in this world.

- First Name Laura
- State/Province WA
- Country USA
- Age   45 - 60
- Type of Yoga do You practice? Vinyasa, Iyengar, Yin
- How long have you practiced Yoga? 2 years, I year consistently

Why do/ did you practice Yoga?

Because nothing beats the total melting relaxation that is savasana! Also, ones find that breathing through discomfort, setting an intention, and becoming stronger and suppler offer many benefits off the mat, too.

- First Name Alice
- State/Province CA
- Country Orange
- Age 45 – 60
- Type of Yoga do You practice? Ashtanga
- How long have you practiced Yoga? 4 years

  Why do/ did you practice Yoga?

Exercise and stress reduction.

- First Name Sharon
- State/Province Rhode Island
- Country USA
- Age 45 - 60
- Type of Yoga do You practice? Amrit
- : How long have you practiced Yoga? 6 years

  Why do/ did you practice Yoga?

I started for health reasons... had a spiritual awakening and now realize how important it is... a way to view the world... meditation in motion.

- First Name Vicky

- State/Province Florida

- Country USA

- Age 30 - 44

- Type of Yoga do You practice? yoga, like the "poses"? I don't do much of that lately to be honest, Troy :) But I guess, much like many say they are Christian and don't see the inside of a church except on holidays... Amrit Yoga.... but I "practice yoga" (as described in the Yoga Sutras) a lot of the time, except when I'm in reaction over some.... well, we won't get into that.

- How long have you practiced Yoga? Again, the "poses" - since Summer of 2013, but otherwise, a whole lot apparently, I just didn't have this particular terminology before I showed up here in the magical forest

Why do/ did you practice Yoga?

It's the only natural way to be, though there are many paths and varieties of lanterns when it gets dark... the other way is chaos, self-deceit and general misery.

- First Name Dorothy

- State/Province Kansas

- Country USA

- Age 45 – 60

- How long have you practiced Yoga? 10

  Why do/ did you practice Yoga?

  It helps me physically, mentally and spiritually all at the same time

- First Name Helene
- State/Province Ca
- Country USA
- Age 30 – 44
- Type of Yoga do You practice? All
- How long have you practiced Yoga? 15 years

Why do/ did you practice Yoga?

It makes me feel more balanced. I sleep better and feel more focused and less stressed.

- First Name Kevin Willis
- State/Province Ca
- Country USA
- Age 45 - 60
- Type of Yoga do You practice? Meditative, Slower-Pace
- How long have you practiced Yoga? Over 1 Year.

  Why do/ did you practice Yoga?

  For personal well-being, mindfulness and awareness - learning techniques to become a better human being.

- First Name Claire

- State/Province Ca

- Country USA

- Age 30 – 44

- Type of Yoga do You practice? Troy's T.E.C. yoga

- How long have you practiced Yoga? 7 years

Why do/ did you practice Yoga?

It helps me live in the moment, deal with life's struggles and frustrations as if they were opportunities for growth, and has lead me to make lifelong friendships along the way.

"Yoga…. Is, everything. Yoga, brings me back to my center, myself, and my happiness. "Sue B.

Dedication

This book is dedicated to all of you who question and search for understanding to this human condition. The students who have also been my teachers that are continually challenging me with questions that I seek out answers too. Hopefully this book will help answer some of your personal questions through the sharing of others' paths of discovery. To my mother and father, my best friends Debbie and Dorothy, to my teachers Diane Ross, Yogi Amrit Desai, Neem Kiroli Baba, Pramahansa Yogananda, Amma, Swami Kripalu, Jesus Christ, Ram Das and my first true teacher and Guru, my brother, Todd E. Cox. I created and named my yoga technique after my brother's initials: Total Engagement Concept.

And these expressions, trials and tribulations shared within could not be possible without the generous sharing, love and journey of the many students who have graced me with their presence along my own journey. Through struggle or great ease, I thank you for the lessons. For they are truly not my students, but my teachers. This book is for you.

I give thanks to all my guides, angels, arc angels, loved one and those on my lineage that have gone before me. May the light bearers who have illuminated my path have their light returned to them in multitudes and may I have the strength to carry their light to others. The light in myself, recognizes the light in you and the point where we merge as one. Namaste!

Y.?.O.G.A.

Idea: Y= The Why? of Yoga; O=Om: Is Yoga a Religion? G=Guru The Importance of Teachers; A= Ascend; Stories of Enlightenment.   This book is the beginning of a series of discourses and investigations into the popularity of yoga. Look for the next book in the series; **The 'O' of Yoga: 'Om' -Is Yoga a Religion?**

Acknowledgments

My light was lit by the torchbearer Diane Ross in 1995. Thorough her continued coaching and encouragement this work is possible. She held the light for me to grow away and come back to the path in my own way. Her continued love and support, advice and inspiration brought me to the way. She has walked with me, holding my hand and loving me without asking for anything in return.

Yogi Amrit Desai, his lineage of masters and the teachings he shares inspired the insights and understandings that lead me to formulate my experiences into thoughts, words, deeds and actions. Karen Adams has worked with me to develop the words and practices that you see here. Her steadfast friendship and willingness to try new ideas and share results, read and edit this work and keep me fresh and unbiased indebted be to her for lifetimes.

Y.?.O.G.A. introduction Mission

Statement of Book

To put the humanity into Yoga and create a unique insight into the current Yoga craze sweeping the U.S. and the globe. To understand the Y? of Yoga; why people are so drawn to this ancient art in its modern incarnation. Why is Yoga so popular? Through the various personal explanations of students' experiences, I will try to find a commonality in why people come together and support each other.

Troy Cox

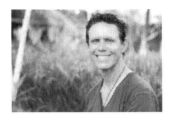

- Amrit Yoga Master Teacher and Yoga Nidra Certified Instructor.
- Creator of 'Sun Salute Yoga' and 'Designer Yoga Teacher Training'.
- Registered 500 Hour ERYT, Yoga Alliance, Master Yoga teacher Amrit Institute.
- Certified by Yogi Amrit Desai, Core Power Yoga, Yoga Fit, AFAA.
- Teaching Yoga for over 13 years, studied meditation 20+ Years.
- Creator of the 'T.E.C.' method. http://www.tecyoga.com
- Published article contributor.
- Developed and leads successful one on one 'Authentic Yoga Teacher Training'.
- Leader of yoga retreats internationally.

Troy Cox Bio:

Master Teacher Troy Cox is the creator of the **Total Engagement Concept™** system. The concept is a natural optimization of all systems of our being technique. It combines the deeper understandings of Yoga philosophy with Personal Training exercise. techniques and Yogic postures, martial arts concepts and movements, mental understanding of Yoga Nidra therapy unblocking the mind, and a detailed approach to structural alignment, with the trainings of the Amrit Method of meditation in motion, leads his students to a 'fine tuning' of all their facilities. Troy's skill at utilizing the posture as a total engagement of our being, and his ability of relating the connection between our physical, mental and inner bodies, leads students to a deeper state of being through techniques he learned that have been handed down from masters from India and Asia. This concept leads students to see how the physical mirrors what is being held mentally and how it affects our higher selves, leading us to unblock and open age old holdings and have deep understanding of ourselves in different reactive states, freeing us from old habits and opening us to new way of being. Total Engagement Concept™, investigates how we relate to the outer world from the inner and our connectedness to all living things. Through his guidance we learn how to allow a divine unity to manifest at last completing who we really are as a whole, totally engaged being, alert and aware in each moment.   As an experience, Total Engagement Concept™ is a series of complex and challenging powerful movements and postures, oral cueing techniques, mentally guided experiences, deep meditative philosophy and Yogic concepts that complete who we truly are, leading us back from the individual to the source of all: One Sun; Many Rays.

Elements

I once was a little boy.
The Sun and Sky were my friends.
Running and playing were my hobbies.
All I wanted was a puppy.

I became a young man traveling the world.
Trials and tribulations were my sometime friends.
Anger and reaction were my hobbies.
All I wanted was commercial success.

Now I am a grown man.
The Sun and the Moon are my loyal companions.
Yoga and Meditation are my lifestyle.
All I want is to merge with the divine.

Troy Cox.

Foreword

"I am honored to have been Troy's first meditation. He didn't know it at the time, but I had learned many of the same meditation techniques that he would also learn through his future yoga teacher, Amrit Desai, whom he met years later. Troy may attribute his success to what he has learned through others, and that is partly true, but his main reason for being so successful is the realization of his authentic self. His journey through his own hells has strengthened him and made him more compassionate, but that's because he chose the path of love and not the path of bitterness. Through his devotion to the path of love, he has shared in this book his concerns for all those who have an interest in yoga. Whether you are a student or a teacher, this book is a must read! This is a rare insight into the world of commercial and private-practice yoga. This is an important book. I urge anyone who has ever thought about taking a yoga class to read every word Troy has written. His authenticity and knowledge of this vast subject combine to bring the reader into an understanding of this ancient art that is extremely valuable. In Troy's own words, *'In the pop yoga world, you will find everything from yoga for abs, butt, thighs, and combined with the latest exercise trends, from ballet to carnival tricks. You can also go the other route and attend spiritual combo events led by dreadlock-headed, pseudo hippies, wearing Indian-themed sarongs that spout a dialog of spiritual soup, that combines every major religion into a love poem that makes everyone feel good. What I am suggesting is that you, as the student, take the time to ask, "why am I here?" What does what is being presented to you have to do with yoga? How is it helping you? What benefits are you receiving? And just to make me happy, is it going to prevent injury? Is it in alignment with our ethics?'*

Troy truly has YOUR best interests at heart. He's not interested in self-promotion or sounding like a teacher. His goal is to keep you safe and connect with your authenticity.

This book not only shares the ins and outs of yoga world, but also shares Troy's heart. I'm sure the reader will come to the same conclusion I did many years ago when I met Troy: He is honest, trustworthy and is a brilliant light unto the world! I am privileged to call him a friend."

Diane L. Ross, author, ***Meditations for Miracles***

"In May, 1977, I was with a small group of American seekers at Kennedy Airport in New York City to welcome Swami Kripalu, a master of Shaktipat Kundalini Yoga from India, for his first visit to the United States. His proposed three-month stay in the United States extended to four years as he found life in the United States conducive to his yoga sadhana.

I stayed with Swami Kripalu during his four-year stay in the United States from 1977-1981 and this changed the trajectory of my life. Due to his influence, I became a yoga practitioner, a yoga teacher, an Ayurvedic Health Care Educator and the author of 16 books, four on the life and teachings of Swami Kripalu.

I decided to donate all royalties from my books on Swami Kripalu to charity as he gave everything to us free with so much joy and love. One of the things I did was to set up the $1000 Swami Kripalu Scholarship (no longer available) at the Amrit Yoga Institute in Salt Springs, Florida to help someone become a yoga teacher.

Troy Cox was our first selection and I couldn't have been more pleased. Not only was Troy a sincere spiritual seeker, but he clearly had an aptitude for yoga.

Following Troy's teacher training, he went on a spiritual pilgrimage to India, returned and founded his own yoga school in California, and now has written his first book on yoga. It is a pleasure to endorse Troy's book, as he writes from the heart about yoga and his own spiritual journey and transformation. It is also a special joy to read his quotes from our beloved Bapuji (Swami Kripalu) who surely has blessed Troy's effort.

Yoga, which means 'union,' is timeless. It was given to the world by the great Masters of India and is a complete road map to self-actualization. Troy's book adds to this wonderful legacy and will be an inspiration to you on your own spiritual journey."

Hari Om Shanti, Shanti, Shanti (May There Be Peace Everywhere)

John Mundahl, author, "The Swami Kripalu Reader: Selected Works from a Yogic Master"
2016

Testimonial

"My experience taking the 200 Hour certified Yoga Teacher Training with Troy was wonderful, challenging and a great enhancement to my personal and professional life. I spent time, nearly two years, researching different yoga teacher training programs. There is an abundance of teacher training programs out there. In the last 5 years I have seen an absolute explosion of programs on the scene. I never found one that I resonated with until I found Troy.

I chose Troy because, first and foremost, of his experience and vast knowledge base. He has taught numerous training programs over the years. He has been in the health and wellness industry over 20 years. He has studied under the tutelage Yogi Amrit Desai and still holds a very close relationship with his teacher. Troy also continues his education and journey by attending many seminars and weekend retreats, which he would readily and generously share with me. Troy's approach is all encompassing and I was exposed to the history and philosophy of yoga. I went into the teacher training program thinking I would master all of the postures. Troy gently and conscientiously guided me through what is the essence of yoga.

The other aspect of Troy's teacher training that I particularly liked was the sequencing of the lectures. We did not jump into the postures right away. We spent much time on the fundamentals of anatomy, physiology and yoga theoretical principals mainly focusing on the yoga sutras, which I thoroughly loved. I told Troy that I could have spent our entire teacher training on the yoga sutras.

Troy is very intelligent, warm, funny and engaging. His knowledge base is incredible. He could answer every question I had whether it be on the yoga sutras, history of yoga, or alternatives to postures to keep myself and students from harm's way. I always felt supported and guided. He is passionate about teaching, yoga, meditation and his students. He offers so much of himself, and is incredibly generous with his knowledge.

I highly recommend taking Troy's 200-hour yoga teacher training program. This program is for people who want to learn about teaching yoga as well as learning about yourself. You will leave feeling prepared to teach classes. You will learn how to use your voice, your body and your mind in ways you did not know were possible. The growth that I experienced I take with me and use on a daily basis. I am forever grateful to Troy and thank him for introducing me to yoga and teaching me the beginning of a lifelong journey."

Samantha Levinson, DPT

Contents

Introduction What is popular Yoga.

"Yoga is popular, what is popular is not Yoga."
-Yogi Amrit Desai

"Everyone has equal claim to yoga and its benefits, but everyone must also observe one primary rule, which is to engage in regular practice. Without practice, even an ordinary task is not accomplished, so how could the extraordinary task of yoga be accomplished? By studying the teaching, a vision of the path may be received, but remember that success does not come in that way. Success comes only through the repeated practice of yoga techniques." **-Swami Kripalavanandaji**

Yoga has become quite a phenomenon in our modern culture today. Especially in the West, where we always tend to look for bigger and better it can be confusing. In the land of opportunity and designer everything you can currently find a style of Yoga to meet your mood for the day. A practitioner, person practicing Yoga, can studio hop from one place to the next on a daily, weekly, monthly basis sampling all the varieties of Yoga out there. With the proliferation of first, coupon sites offering classes for as low as one dollar a day to the now popular membership app downloads that let you attend multiple studios offering everything from spin bike Yoga to Barre classes, one can never have to lock into a particular style of Yoga. Choices range from Yoga in the park, stand up paddle board yoga, trampoline yoga, Kundalini, Ashtanga, Hatha, Power, Hot, Yin, Restorative, Acrobatic, rope, silk banner Yoga; the list goes on and on. Studios pop up every day on the Yoga scene from giant

Yoga corporation studios to private owned studios. One can take a Yoga retreat to far off exotic locals like Bali or Argentina or in Sedona or Ojai. There are Yoga trainings happening in garages or huge schools and centers. One can join an association such as Yoga Alliance to become a

'registered' teacher or do it underground since the industry is not regulated. Pretty much, anyone can become a Yoga teacher with little to no training.

People doing Yoga come in all shapes and sizes from ex hippies to hippie wannabes, from $300 designer outfitted (not including cost of mat) fitness models to nearly naked hot bodies sweating it out in sauna yoga studios. Chain and corporate studios dubbed 'Mc Yoga' has sprung up everywhere and taken root in our culture. Historically, one used to have to seek out a guide that had studied for years, maybe even in India if you were lucky, and move into an Ashram to learn the true ways of Yoga. Nowadays, Yoga secrets are offered up in pop culture Yoga lifestyle magazines filled with advertisements for everything to the latest designer water to trendy clothes, from celebrities or rock star, sponsored festival circuit Yogis.

No longer a passing fad, it is here to stay in one form or another. But what does it all mean? Where does it come from? How do we know what path is right for us without becoming stressed out by our distressing Yoga? Is it a religion? What is the right way to do a posture? What if I am not flexible? Do I have to meditate? Why do I feel so much better at the end? As a Yoga instructor of twelve plus years and a meditation student of 21 plus years, these are all questions I have asked and have had my students present. My intention for this book is to share some of the answers to all the questions that my students and I have found. I hope to shed a light on this popular and profit making machine called Yoga through my personal experience, my seeking of answers and deeper meanings and those my students have shared with me. I also intend to share my insight of Yoga principals and philosophies in a formula that I know works so you can find your answers to the questions you may have.

Yoga is a multi-Billions dollar a year industry. Yes, that's a Billions. How could it all be helpful? So many students come to me after feeling lost or being hurt and misguided. I have heard stories of students being mishandled so brutally that they lay down their mats forever and never intend to return. I have been a studio owner and led teacher trainings, hired and let go of teachers, seen the business of Yoga in a studio setting and on a corporate level. I have heard direct accounts from other studio owners and festival producers of the unspoken side of Yoga and teachers, which I will expand on in the chapter Why Not to Do Yoga. I have traveled and tried to take a class from all the top American Yoga teachers. Through years of coaching and hearing these stories and more I have seen a need for help in determining what it is you may need to be receiving from Yoga as a new student beginning your practice, or a seasoned professional looking for a way to guide your student. I am brutally honest in my information and do not believe in glossing over or sweeping under the rug.

Make the time to take as many different styles of Yoga that call out to you. It is easy to get locked into one style and think that is Yoga. Yoga is indefinable. It, to me, is a martial art, a discipline. It takes fortitude, practice, experience and passion. There are so many styles of 'Yoga' being invented every year here in America. You could go your whole life learning. What I think you will find, is one style will be 'Your Style' for a while, maybe months, maybe years, then you will evolve into something else. This way you are climbing a ladder of Yoga.

I don't think it is beneficial to 'Guru Hop' where you take one class from this person and that. I think it is good to see if a style calls to you and then get absorbed in it as much as you can. When it no longer satisfies see what the next progression would be. My Guru has a saying; "Yoga is popular, what is popular is NOT Yoga." I see this in all the trends and 'new' ways of doing Yoga. While it is fantastic that Yoga is exploding in our culture where it is much needed, one should ask, why they are doing Yoga? What is the perceived result desired from this form or practice? Is standing on my head on an unstable board in the ocean really going to benefit my journey? What is the reason you are on your Yoga path? Why are you there?

If the teacher, style, presentation of information, lifestyle, morals, ethics, heck, even the music are not serving your higher good, why endure?

As my first meditation teacher says in her book 'Meditations for Miracles.' "The only virtue in suffering is realizing that you do not need to suffer." I do not relate to boot camp style training or the drill sergeant; you must be in pain to gain, mentality. I do believe in discipline but that is an entirely different lesson than being demeaned and in pain. If you are taking a style of Yoga or what is being called Yoga, ask yourself how it is serving you and your greatest good. That is the purpose of Yoga, the design of this system of eight limbs is to serve the evolution of all mankind. Inherent in the foundation tracing back thousands of years is the idea of maximizing one's human experience on all planes of existence. To reduce suffering and separation and create unity and oneness is the definition of the word Yoga, Yog, to Yoke or draw out your maximum potential. How can you create unity when you are in an uncomfortable situation, in stress without knowing why you are there?

If you are new to Yoga, experienced or just checking it out to see if you want to do it, why is the beginning. Each posture should be for a purpose, a reason, physical, mental, energetic, psychic, emotional, and awareness. Tell me what your intention is? No really, what is it you want from what you are doing? What are you doing and what are you getting out of it? I ask this several times in class as a leader. Mostly I get blank stares. How can we know what we want if we don't know who we are or what we truly hope to get out of something? Have you ever felt blindly led into a situation without knowing why you are there and then left with a feeling of being lost? This does not just apply to Yoga, we all do it all the time. Whether you never pick up a Yoga mat or try a class, you can use these guide posts I have created to determine exactly what it is you want and how to get it now. If you are considering Yoga or currently practicing, this self-exploration can create instant clarity for you on your path.

What is this Yoga thing everyone seems to be talking about? How do you start, or if you are started, how to proceed? Just the word Yoga can be daunting, let alone the pretext, deeper meanings, esoteric understandings and reasons for doing it. If you are like me, you thought it was something foreign, maybe a religion, or just a form of exercise. But if everyone else is doing it, there must be something to it, right? It must be something worth checking into. However, there is one catch. You must know what it is you want *first* before entering. Your intention must be clear or you could be lost in the sea of modern Yoga. Its confusing out there and you can waste time and energy by not knowing how to start or where to go.

This book will guide you through the maze with the help of my students, teachers and personal experiences from a teacher's perspective but more importantly, help you determine what you want so your path is clear through a specific formula. We will set the guide posts for you, it will take action on your part, but we can illuminate your torch so you can see down the path you decide to choose.

The money machine we now call yoga in the west is no longer a cottage industry but a mega financial product complete with corporatization, legal actions and teachers trying to patent postures. Misinformation and well intentioned instructors are leading student and seekers into perilous pits of danger and injury. My mission has always been to keep others safe, especially anyone who is seeking my council or drawing on my experience. I believe that safety first will keep us out of trouble or from getting hurt. This is not working from the fear of getting hurt, rather the strong desire within myself to approach life from an informed and educated position. I believe that education can bring about World peace (Shanti, my Yogic namesake). My hope is that through my experience and research I can help anyone seeking potential answers and health benefits by making this Yoga industry transparent. Often times we would rather have things unpleasant hidden. It makes things easier to digest. Personally, I need to know the rules and the pitfalls before I feel ready to enter into a new venture. This is for those that feel the same way.

Don't worry, there are no worksheets, no homework, no one handing out passes or fail, but you do have to be honest and brave. Through this journey together we will dispel myths and misperceptions, avoid potential danger and come out at the end of the path with clarity and light around your life and the reason for what you are doing. You will no longer enter into situations without knowing why you are there and what you are supposed to be getting. You just need to be willing to take the steps forward, we have laid out where the traps are, trust yourself, you can do it and will come out on the other side with a sense of union, all systems functioning optimally.

My journey did not begin with Yoga. It began with seeking answers to life's greatest mystery. Is there anything after death? I needed to know that this thing called life was for something. Not just aimlessly roaming the planet, doing as we please, seeking material satisfaction. After the passing of my little brother in 1994 in a horrible motorcycle vehicular manslaughter that took both his life and the life of his girlfriend, the mother of two and watching the illegal, unlicensed driver walk free of charges, my life shattered and fell apart. I did not know who I was anymore or what was important. I was a very popular radio personality and mobile party D.J. in Kansas City. I had artfully survived the transition from the oldest A.M. rock and roll radio station being bought out and transitioned into the perfect format for my voice, adult contemporary. I partied on the weekends with people for pay at weddings, birthdays and graduations. I was ego driven and consumed with becoming a famous radio host like Ryan Seacrest, only in my age it was Dick Clark who was my hero. From radio to T.V. hosting to fame was my path. I dated whomever I please, drank and ran my mouth a lot.

I tried to return to that life again after burying my brother, but I could no longer function as I had. Everything felt so hollow and meaningless. So I ran away to the Florida Keys and disappeared from reality for a year and a half on a private island. After much mourning, I was ready to reemerge into society. I began a spiritual quest for answers. I read one book on every major religion that I could find. My therapist finally gave me the choice, take a prescription anti-depressant or find a meditation teacher. This led me to meet my first meditation teacher, Diane Ross. She saved me from a dark path I was heading down that could have led to self-destructive behaviors. I studied with her for ten years while recreating my materialistic radio and D.J. life I had been living before.

I moved to California to pursue my dreams of acting and being a T.V. host. Ryan Seacrest had just premiered in front of the world on American Idol. I knew I could do it too. Back in a stressful, competitive environment in one of the largest cities of the world I was able to work with some of the meditation techniques she gave me to avoid stress and had great success within my first two years gaining union status and having two agents. However, I felt hollow and empty still. There had to be more to life. I had more to give to others that would help them in their searching. That realization led me to leave L.A. and continue my soul searching.

I had been working out since I was a scrawny 17-year-old, tired of being picked on. I decided to use my life's knowledge of healthy eating and exercise, and begin a new career as a Personal Trainer. While working on my certification I decided I should complement my income with something related to body building but in a group situation. A friend suggested I try a Yoga class, that with my theatrical and radio experience, I might be a good teacher. Being the only male was awkward, but not as much as not being able to touch my toes or lift my arms over head. All I had ever done was lift heavy weight, especially now at this place I was at in my life. I was grunting through the postures and really not enjoying it, feeling like a bull in a china shop when something happened. Suddenly, my meditation training kicked in and before I knew it the class was over. It was as if I had floated through all the postures. I was amazed an hour had passed. I felt so calm. I thought meditation could only happen lying down with the lights off, some soft music and incense burning. It had never occurred to me that you could move and meditate.

After completing my first training I worked for two years as a Personal Trainer before starting to consider teaching Yoga. I wanted to take as many classes as I could to find out more about it. I took the second level of Yoga Fit's teacher training program and continued attending classes with the most popular teachers in L.A. After all, if they were on magazines and in L.A., they must know something about the experience I had. Once I had the courage to try and teach my first class I remember still feeling like I knew nothing. The first time on the microphone, in front of a group all looking at me was a nerve wracking experience. I still remember shaking, sweating and doing the entire class with my back to the room. My theatrical training did no good as I stood at the front and just hoped everyone could see me and follow along to the one routine I had memorized. I am certain, now in retrospect, that it was awful. What is worse is I know I taught that same format, at the front of the room, with my back to the class, for the next year or longer.

My acting and voice training had always paid off, so I know I sounded OK, I knew how to perform the postures, but I knew nothing about teaching. I was still weight lifting, so body building was still my passion and I hit the gym more than I was doing Yoga. But slowly, I started to notice differences in my body. The first thing I noticed was my tension headaches starting to subside. Then over time, I could touch my toes. I started noticing I was happier and less sore after lifting weights. I was starting to unconsciously feel the effects of Yoga on my body. This was a door way. It started to lead me inward. So I retook my original level one training and then enrolled in level three Yoga Fit training. Still obsessed with fitness, I did not have any interest in the spiritual side of Yoga, only how it could keep helping my body and others.

Level three training was a little surprise. The group was nice, and we touched on the deeper stuff in Yoga briefly, but I noticed the staff was distant and I met the owner of Yoga Fit. I think I brushed her the wrong way and I took a step back and realized that I was being taught fitness and tight bun and strong core routines, but no one was wanting to talk about the strange meditative trance I went into in my first class and I was being sold a bunch of merchandise. My eyes were opened and it was my first look at Yoga as a business model. I was just learning a workout. There had to be a different approach but no one was talking about it.

I kept teaching gym Yoga and eventually got into and went to three Core Power Hot Yoga trainings. I had been teaching for five years at this point and I heard so many good stories from my students about the way Yoga was benefiting them. For me, my headaches had stopped and I was calmer. Sure the benefits of Yoga were evident and we learned a little about them as a side note in the trainings. I found the Hot Yoga world even less spiritual or meditative. I became obsessed with Bikram Yoga and knew that he must have designed it like the military to wear you down until you had to break through to some understanding. Corporate Yoga teaching was extremely competitive and after being coldly and impersonally let go for a scheduling misunderstanding on Christmas Eve, I decided I wanted to learn more about "real" Yoga, but from an authentic source. No more chain American Franchise Yoga for me.

Researching Yogis living in America I narrowed it down to two. One, Deepak Chopra was very close, the second, Yogi Amrit Desai was far away in Florida. So I went to the Chopra Center in Encinitas and dragged along three of my gym Yoga students. I took time after class to speak with the teacher, after all the ladies stopped fawning over him, and told him my quest. He let me know the other Indian teacher; Amrit Desai was making a rare West Coast appearance in two weeks. I was excited to get to meet a real Yogi from India; he must know the answer to what had happened to me in my first Yoga class. I was also skeptical and nervous. My family roots are in Kansas and there are two things I was always told to stay away from, snake oil salesmen and hippies.

So much has happened since that first class of his I took. I can truly say I am a completely different person, but essentially the same. A better man has grown out of what I thought I was. Sitting in the far back of a giant ball room in Los Angeles with my seventy-year-old friend and personal training client waiting for the Indian teacher to come out was so comical to me. It was everything foreign and not in my realm of Yoga. Some students were all dressed in white, some in traditional Indian Saris. No one but my friend and I had a Yoga mat. They all had bolsters and blankets. I was ready to run. Too much fanfare, finally the man I had seen on the internet, Amrit Desai, entered the room. I almost rolled my eyes in the pomp and circumstance and the strange prayers and chanting. There had been none of that in my eight fitness and hot Yoga teacher trainings. This was strange to me. But he seemed loved and his talk was very loving. He seemed harmless to me. I noticed as I sat I wanted to go into my meditation trainings. I tried to stay present. Then the strangest thing happened to me.

Thirty minutes into his talk a muscle spasm started in my forehead. Not on my forehead, but inside my skull. It was like an eye twitch, but from the inside out. I went to the restroom to look at my forehead and see why it was twitching. As I stared in the mirror, nothing was moving. I still felt the twitch, but no muscles were moving. I was mystified. I went back to hear the guru's talk and the twitching intensified. Before I knew it I was at the table at the end of the talk signing up for training in Florida and offering to drive him to his next location in San Diego. My friend with me thought it was amazing. We really had no idea who he was; we just both had the desire to be closer to him.

Four years later, Yogi Amrit Desai came to my Yoga studio, Sun Salute Yoga, for 'The Urge to Merge' workshop. It was a day of bliss. As I sat and looked at his photo that I always have out, and looked over to the right where he was sitting, I was tickled with bliss. My now Guru, who has illuminated my life and explained so much about Yoga's true meanings was back in California speaking to my students. Full circle. Four years ago, I did not know I could grin from ear to ear. I was still lost in the missing parts. But now I felt whole again. I watched as others would laugh out loud at Gurudev's mix of insight and humor (oh God, let all my Guru's have a sense of humor). I was thrilled to see others taking notes, hearing the truth in the message. I delighted when others eyes glimpsed over at me and twinkled as he answered their questions.

I floated on a cloud I thought was a cushion under me as I looked up at my teacher. No saint, but a man. This was a man who faced some real challenges on his path and endured life's ups and downs but stayed in the light of love and returned to the teaching of Yoga. My heart bursts at the seams, when I think of how I have grown, knowing this system is possible for all. This is what life was supposed to be about. I was so proud he was in the Yoga studio and that his teachings allowed me to create. He was my alter to truth, light and love that I now offer up to the world. I glided out the door as the day wound down and hugged him goodbye in the rain. I bravely said, 'I love you Gurudev'. My light exploded in ecstasy as he said 'I love you too', back to me. Oh God, thank you for your teachers, Oh God, thank you for my brother, Oh God thank you for showing me the light of your love. Satnam; Truth is we are meant to live a life of light and love. Oft' times, we need to be reminded and sometimes those reminders are hard to survive, but survive we must, to shine on.

I have since fallen in love with Yoga and all the medical benefits it offers. I have facilitated multiple teacher trainings and have teachers teaching regularly. I have continued taking teacher trainings from famous and well known American teachers, gone back to hot Yoga, Yoga festivals and explored the vast world of Yoga. My students are still getting great results for injuries and for weight loss just to name a few of the benefits. I kept noticing that I am feeling better and slowly becoming calmer.

It has become my mission to educate myself as much in Western and authentic Eastern Yoga and infusing this knowledge into my own teachings. It is what I want to do more than anything and it will help me and others for the rest of my life. I have ridden the wave of ups and downs owning the number one Yoga Studio in town for five years. When the city announced it was going to tear down our building for rezoning, we closed our doors. With the growing and unfair popularity of illegal donation based yoga not following the legal guidelines of a donation for profit business or employment laws it was an easy decision to follow the signs. I decided I needed to pursue being a student again for my own growth. Closing the studio has propelled me into a deeper investigation of the modern popularity of yoga that has swept the world in the last few decades. The day to day operations of owning a business and providing for my students and teachers needs has been replaced with a burning desire to understand why so many others are turning to yoga as the answer to our chaotic modern world. In order to grow I again needed to learn. It is my hope that this learning, will become your learning, answering a wide net of questions about why you should try safe, smart Yoga.

CHAPTER ONE
Why do Yoga?

"When the mind returns to where your body is, when the mind is doing what your body is doing, when you mind is totally focused on what your body is feeling, when your thoughts, feeling and actions are moving as one, you merge into the integrative experience of Yoga."

-*Yogi Amrit Desai*

"We insult the science of yoga if we think that its techniques are only useful in curing disease. One can cut vegetables with a sword, but a sword's potential is wasted if it is used only for cutting vegetables. It is more accurate to say that yoga contains the tools for true self-development." -

Swami Kirpalavanandaji

Yoga for all ages

There is yoga for everyone now. Yoga for kids, lots of fun, meowing to cat pose and mooing to cow. Some counties still keep yoga separated from the education system for fear it's a religion. Postures are not a religion, at best they are a release of stress at worse a stretch class. Most yoga today is made accessible to all. Yoga for seniors, water aerobics yoga, post-traumatic stress syndrome yoga, yoga for runners, swimmers, athletes, yoga for stopping smoking, there is a version of yoga for all types. One just has to research a little and take the correct class for their needs and limitations. When the medical world started to recommend yoga to their students and put it on its way to being covered by insurance, we all rejoiced. However, most doctors thought all yoga was the same.

A vigorous class taught for exercise benefits. So they would recommend someone recovering to not do yoga. I would always advise to listen to your doctor when making any decisions. Opinion and education have changed since then and now it is becoming better understood that there is a type of yoga for all types. One just has to do some research and look into the styles and types. That is one reason for this book. I would like anyone who is interested in the health benefits of yoga to feel they could try a class and see if it helps them safely.

Long before I knew about Yoga I was a lifeguard at a YWCA in downtown Kansas City. Personally I was just interested in getting off work to use the weights and machines to get bigger. What I remember the most is the seventy and eighty-year old's. Every morning at 6 a.m. sharp with a second shift arriving at 7 a.m. a small group of seniors would come in to the pool with a smile and wave. They did not all walk that well with various limps and waddles, but once they got in the water they became the most graceful water creatures ever imagined. It was like that movie Cocoon. They swam and swam in a straight line for an hour and some an hour and half at a time with nary a stop. Little rubber swim caps bobbing up and down in a straight line. Lithe arms with paper thin skin reaching and reaching and reaching through the water like it was nothing. Here I was a muscle bound twenty something and I couldn't lift my arm over my head for five minutes without my shoulders killing me, let alone breast stroke for an hour without stopping. That made such a huge impression on me of the importance of movement and the human body as we age. The body can do miraculous things. But the one thing it was made to do was to move. Here they were, living proof that if you move you keep healthy and strong. And with a wave and a smile too. I will always be inspired by that morning crew of senior swimmers.

I remember meeting Caroline the first day. She was my first personal training client over fifty years old and she did not like me calling her a senior. I remember she said: '*I am not the age of my body, I am the age of my mind and I am youthful in my mind.*' Sitting before me on a bench. My manager at the gym thought she would be a good client for me since I taught Yoga and really needed to stretch. I saw in her eyes a glimmer of wide eyed wonder. I have always been able to see into people. I see a light or a glimmer like a doorway in. However there usually lies in most, a conflict between the potential I see and the reality they are living. She was wearing large sweat pants, big white nurse type shoes and several layers of shirts a sweater and a fleece jacket. She needed help to sit and stand on her own with me holding her arms. Yet I could see an eagerness in her eyes. It was as if I could see a little girl of 12 or 14 trapped inside an experienced person's body. I knew the work I had been doing as a Yoga teacher would work best with this client more than personal training workouts. I knew the most important work we would need to do was overcoming fear. It was several sessions in before I had the courage to ask her about her appearance. What she said broke my heart but reaffirmed the challenge I had given myself to really work with this individual to the end result, no matter the price it would cost me. 'When you reach a certain age, you don't want to look in the mirror because what looks back is not how you see yourself in your mind. So I don't look in the mirror.'

The work with her has been both rewarding and challenging. Fear is the hardest to deal with and resolve. Harder than changing the body. As we worked through the program I developed, her body responded surprisingly quickly. She gained confidence, saw a hairdresser and lost our goal pounds. As her confidence grew, she purchased new clothes and looked for a social group of women. I used yoga principals of observation and mindfulness techniques to help her overcome some of the fear she had. We worked on postures that I just called stretches but were yoga postures. I remember the first time I put the aerobic step down in the middle of the cardio room away from the wall. I looked around the room and saw other people working out looking out of the corners of their eyes as this senior client was crying and trembling. I felt awful as she processed her fear and had a panic attack. But having worked with my Yoga students I knew that they had overcome their fear of difficult postures with a technique I had developed. Through my method of combining certain yoga techniques in an order I had developed, much progress was made over fear and self-confidence. She was so happy with her progress that she accompanied me on a trek across the country to study with Amrit Desai. We worked together for seven years. In that time when Carol got healthy enough to have double knee replacement surgery, lost 65 pounds, gets around well, laughs, has girlfriends, a social life, gets out and is engaged again in life. She was the only person I wanted to take with me when I found the Yoga teacher in L.A. and she went along gladly. Her age did not matter in her transformation, as she made it clear to me on our first meeting, she is not her age. My approach to yoga awoke something in her and she changed her life's experience.

I figured she would be discerning in her opinion and I could trust her advice in my wanting to find the right teacher to learn more about the depth of Yoga. And I thought I could share with the teacher my greatest success story through Yoga. We got to meet him and actually volunteered to drive him all the way to San Diego. There was my client in the front seat giggling like a little girl asking the guru questions. He sat in the back and obliged her questions and made observations about how beautiful Southern California is. While at a bathroom break I shared with him Carol's success story. He was delighted to hear about her transformation. I felt such calmness in his presence and my third eye buzzed for days after. Before I knew it Carol and I were flying across the country to the Guru's ashram to learn mediation from him. Although she has thanked me over and over for working with her, but it is truly I that owe her gratitude. For she has shown me that through working with the darkest part of fear in our mind we can get through it when someone else knows when to hold our hand and when to let go and believe in us. Through overcoming blocks in our mind and miss beliefs about our capabilities, we can overcome all types of obstacles, both physical and mental. By working with the breath to calm the nervous system, then allowing any reactions to rise and pass instead of trying to stuff them down and watching them after to see if they were real fears of life and death or misperceptions of the mind we can overcome our greatest fears. If she had let age hold her back, she would not have had this revitalization in her life. Yoga is for all ages.

I invite a dialog about what Yoga is, through the ages and in a modern context. I see yoga as an acronym. The acronym stands for the idea that you have to open up to the inner guru to ascend. I always start class by asking the student what their intention is? Ask yourself what your intention is right now. No really, what is it you want from what you are doing? What are you doing and what are you getting out of it? I ask this several times in class as a leader. Mostly I get blank stares. How can we know what we want if we don't know who we are or what we truly hope to get out of something? Have you ever felt blindly led into a situation without knowing why you are there and then left with a feeling of being lost? This does not just apply to Yoga, we all do it all the time. Weather you never pick up a Yoga mat or try a class, you can use these guide posts I have created to determine exactly what it is you want and how to get it now. If you are considering Yoga or currently practicing, this self-exploration can create instant clarity for you on your path.

What is this Yoga thing everyone seems to be talking about? How do you start, or if you are started, how to proceed? Just the word Yoga can be daunting, let alone the pretext, deeper meanings, esoteric understandings and reasons for doing it. If you are like me, you thought it was something foreign, maybe a religion, or just a form of exercise. But if everyone else is doing it, there must be something to it, right? It must be something worth checking into. However, there is one catch. You must know what it is you want first before entering. Your intention must be clear or you could be lost in the sea of modern Yoga. Its confusing out there and you can waste time and energy by not knowing how to start or where to go. This book will guide you through the maze with the help of my students, teachers and personal experiences from a teacher's perspective but more importantly, help you determine what you want so your path is clear through a specific formula. We will set the guide posts for you, it will take action on your part, but we can illuminate your torch so you can see down the path you decide to choose.

Yoga has become quite a phenomenon in our modern culture today. Especially in the West, where we always tend to look for bigger and better it can be confusing. In the land of opportunity and designer everything you can currently find a style of Yoga to meet your mood for the day. A practitioner (person practicing Yoga) can studio hop from one place to the next on a daily, weekly, monthly basis sampling all the varieties of Yoga out there. Yoga in the park, stand up paddle board yoga, trampoline yoga, Kundalini, Ashtanga, Hatha, Power, Hot, Yin, Restorative, the list goes on and on. Studios pop up every day on the Yoga scene from giant Yoga corporation studios to private owned studios. One can take a Yoga retreat to far off exotic locals like Bali or Argentina or even without leaving the country in Sedona or Ojai to name a few places. There are Yoga trainings happening in garages or huge schools and centers. One can join an association such as Yoga Alliance or do it underground since the industry is not regulated. Yogis come in all shapes and sizes from ex hippies to hippie wannabes, from $300 designer outfitted (not including cost of mat) fitness models to nearly naked hot bodies sweating it out in sauna yoga studios. Mc Yoga has sprung up everywhere and taken root in our culture. No longer a passing fad, it is here to stay in one form or another. But what does it all mean? Where does it come from? How do we know what path is right for us without becoming stressed out by our distressing Yoga? Is it a religion? What is the right way to do a posture? What if I am not flexible? Do I have to meditate? Why do I feel so much better at the end? As a Yoga instructor of eleven years and a meditation student of 19 years these are all questions I have asked and have had my students present. My intention for this book is to share some of the answers to all the ?'s that my students and I have found. I hope to shed a light on this machine called Yoga through my personal experience, my seeking of answers and deeper meanings and those my students have shared with me. I also intend to share my insight of Yoga principals and philosophies in a formula that I know works so you can find your answers to the ?'s you may have.

Community

A Yoga room is a room full of a variety of people, all ages and sizes facing forward on rubber mats wearing workout clothes waiting for the teacher to enter. He or She enters and says nice things to the students, calling some by name, chatting in a friendly manner or they enter silently to the front without a word. The teacher has the class start in posture, then they instruct everyone to breath and quote something positive and uplifting. They instruct us to remember that there is no competition in Yoga except with ourselves. The teacher then leads the class through a variety of postures for 60 minutes or 90 minutes with various references to breathe, affirmations, body alignment and occasionally make adjustments on the students. Everyone looks different in each posture, no two the same. The class slows down and ends laying down prone listening to some soft music or silence and the teacher instructs to try to be still and not even think. After a few moments the teacher has the students sit up in a crossed legged position and breath together being grateful and then everyone says Namaste together. Some students get up and roll up their mat silently and gather their belongings, some stay and talk and chat and the energy is buzzing between them, some go to talk to the teacher. For the most part, that is Yoga in the modern world for us Westerners.

For sixty minutes or ninety, if you're lucky, the world disappears. You become a scientist, exploring and discovering new things about yourself. The teacher is instructing you to notice the breath, feel the posture, align your joints, feel the tightness of your ligaments holding the body together. You may feel frustrated that that person next to you can to a seemingly perfect posture but you can't keep your arms over your head. Surely you can do a pushup, but the Yoga pushup is something weird. But some of the shapes the teacher is requesting, are easy for you. Ha! You can to that backbend, but the other person couldn't. You must be better at this stuff than you thought. By the end of the class you note that not only are these your experiences but you hear others in the room talking about how Yoga has helped them. Suddenly your part of a community of likeminded people you did not even know you had. The daily boredom is gone; it just leaves after a while. You can finally BE. Nothing else is in mind but total balance and your coached to be fully present for the first time in memory. As the teacher speaks the student's minds soften. You are asked to be fully engaged, activated, learning and more importantly experiencing. The minds boredom just leaves, boredom with life, with career, with others, with the mundane and ordinary the mind becomes bored with the scope of the global politics and world economy slowly slips away.

Mental Focus

One teaching point made repetitively by a mentor and teacher of mine whose name is Chandrakant, "When I asked you to notice the content of your mind, were you thinking of your name, your age, your job, your sex?" Chandrakant the teacher asks the room of students after leading them into a simple exercise of energy follows attention by guiding them through breathing exercise and through their body. 'I was thinking of how heavy my arm felt holding it up' one student replies. "So when I asked you to notice the content of your mind, was there a gap between my questions and when you thought your arm felt heavy?" The student thinks for a minute and replies "Yes I guess there was, just a short one." The teacher replies with "Exactly, that's what I am concerned with, that gap, in that gap, were you thinking of your name, your age, your sex, your identity?" 'No' says the student, seemingly entranced with their own answer. In that moment, in that Gap, that is Yoga, union, no separation, one with all and one within at the same time. This is the entire point of Yoga in one brief and concise moment. The challenge becomes once we experience that moment; how do we maintain that union?

You will hear two very much quoted lines from Yoga teachers in just about every situation. Yoga means 'Union' and Yoga is 'Modification of the mind stuff.' I'm on the cusp of great success and growth. Or dramatic failure and sadness. I chose to believe the first statement wholeheartedly. Although the other voice creeps in at times, I allow it to exist as doubt is a part of being human and the voice of fear which we all have. That's doesn't mean it is true. What we believe we empower. One of my Guru's instructions for Yoga Nidra is to notice how energy follows attention. That which we focus our attention on attracts our energy. Try it now. Focus on the tip of your nose. Let all other thoughts dissolve and only think about the very tip of your nose. Try it now.

I bet before I asked you to focus on your nose, you were happily unaware of your nose. Then it became clear that all you could think about was that finite point of your nose as all your energy rushed there.

This principle works the same with thoughts. As the thought of successes comes to mind it is usually shadowed by fear. If we acknowledge the fear and release it, returning all our attention on the feeling of successes our energy will flow in that direction. So when looking at yoga, use the approach of watching to see what responds in your body.

Physical Strength

Yoga can get a student to recruit the smaller muscles in the body that lead to joint stability and strength. These muscles are sometimes never even felt by the owner of the body. Most of the time the body uses the largest mover muscles to do the work when we move throughout the day. The support groups are usually never recruited in normal day to day activity. Yoga can teach one to use the support muscles and gain strength in areas such as around joints. Thereby balance can improve when there are not preexisting medical reasons for balance loss.

Flexibility and strength go hand in hand. As a student strengthens and feels the added support of the support muscles and joints, they begin to naturally walk taller. Their posture improves. Sometimes even those with painful arthritis have noted improvement in flexibility and less pain. The encouragement I give my students is to find a teacher who specializes in certain conditions or have been trained to deal with special areas of interest, just like medical specialists. There are many teachers who tout the benefits of yoga as they are taught to say in their training but have not been trained in a specialist area. I can assist with many needs, but a medical diagnosis is another endeavor. I always advise that the doctor is right. No matter what I may think or suggest, the doctor's opinion comes first.

Male students are typically great at the strength poses while the flexibility poses a challenge. I find a lot of fun in talking to other guys or men about yoga. There still remain so many stereo types about the art of yoga. So many times a conversation with a guy will sound like this: "I tried Yoga once and it was so hard and I am just not flexible that I never went back. It kicked my ass dude. I was kind of embarrassed because I couldn't do anything. I can't even touch my toes man. I hurt so much the next day I couldn't believe it. All the girls were doing like these crazy postures. I thought it was going to be easy but I couldn't do Jack. So I gave my mat away. It's just not for me. I'm so not flexible." This is a typical conversation I have with most guys. I couldn't touch my toes when I started either. All I did was lift weights. But now I feel great. You just have to pick the right class. Stay with gentle yoga and work from there. Guys are typically tighter and better at strength poses.

Most guys would rather go out and get on a piece of fiberglass and throw themselves down a rocky cliff covered in powder or slam a head against the reef in a wetsuit over taking a yoga class. I was a body builder and went from not touching my toes with shoulders so tight I couldn't hold my arms over my head for sixty seconds without excruciating pain to twelve years later doing the splits and putting my foot behind my head. Believe me it wasn't easy. I got in there, often the only guy, and worked my ass off. I took every kind of Yoga out there. I suffered injuries from pushing too far. I had to take time off to heal and go back. Yes, I even had to stop lifting so heavy at the gym. Sometimes I felt like some kind of tall weirdo in the yoga room that couldn't do anything. But I did it. And the results are that I'm less wired, my joints move and don't ache, I can breathe deeply, people comment on how calm I seem and I feel great. My last check up with a medical professional was eight or so years ago and the doctor said if it wasn't for what I was doing I would be on blood pressure and cholesterol medication because of my DNA. So I keep doing what I was doing. I never get sick and have more energy than ever.

Most students are first attracted to the glamor of postures. Acro Yoga is a great example. Flashy postures and lifts with two people. It is alluring, fun to watch, physically strenuous and a great workout. People spin it as Yoga because you have to really work with the partner, creating a type of union. Union is a great catch word tossed around a bit. It really means something entirely different than what we think, but more on that later. Working hard and achieving a goal is inherently bred into most of us as a way of life. The harder you work the better chance you have of success. However fun it is to work on a challenging posture and then look for the next challenge, postures are only one part of the puzzle called Yoga. My friend, fellow yoga teacher and fire spinning artist Claire tell me that usually fire and LED lighted tools are the sparkle that attracts people to the spinning arts, and that is great for new artist, but then one wants to develop their skills and focus on the artistry. The same applies for Yoga. Postures are the sparkle that attract new students, but the real skills come later.

Your body is beautiful just the way it is. You have a powerful set of functioning organs. Our bodies are meant to move, and move a lot. They are meant to exercise and move every day. Now exercise does not just mean going the gym and lifting weights. Exercise and move in ways like vacuuming, to walking around the neighborhood, to playing catch with the kids. You don't have to be inside on a machine or lifting dumbbells to get exercise. But how much time do we have to invest in this exercise? So if you are not doing any or all of the above you may need to time crunch and get the most out of your exercise time by taking a high intensity class.

If the body is not moved it will lose its range of motion over time, slow down and ache. Most signs of aging are rated by a loss of flexibility in the muscle, mobility in the joints, and weight gain. All of this can be prevented or minimized through preventive measures. Combined with a healthy diet, the body's weight can be minimized or stalled by consistent exercise. The brain which regulates balance and stability is challenged by consistent learning. Nothing can challenge the mind more than learning new balance and coordination challenging ways of moving. This flow of growth and its effect on the mind will help to increase passion for life and improvement of mood. What comes to you is what you are putting out. The stronger your heart and lungs are, the stronger your blood oxygen ratio is, the stronger your organs work together for health. The more we move and stretch the body, the more improvements we will see. This is true for any form of exercise, especially Yoga. However, the real results come from moving past the postures.

Improved Cardiovascular Health

One of the major components of Yoga is practicing inward focus and attention on one's self. The result is the rising of energy in the practitioner. If you are more of a scientific mind you may wish to call it electrical activity. Electricity runs the body. When we learn techniques, such as Pranayama or breath control, one may sense that it is easier to sense the energy, or Prana, flowing through the body. Prana and Pranayama are two separate but codependent elements. Begin to notice how you feel prior to class and after. Notice if your energy feels elevated. The more you are on the Yoga path, the more tools you will find to help you develop awareness of the energy of life. Just as Yoga has manifested in countless schools and styles in the world, so have techniques to increase and flow energy. You can spend your whole life studying such topics as Kundalini Yoga, Tantric Yoga, Pranayama and still just scratch the surface of energy building tools that are available. Yoga can begin your journey of working with your own energy awareness, and your level of energy expenditure and storage. Think of the physiology of the body and how the energy system is designed. Our anatomy runs on energy or oxygen. The element of oxygen is a gas. It is colorless, tasteless, odorless and gaseous and yet we depend on its existence. The lungs capture it even though we normally have little awareness of it. Oxygen is then pumped into our blood stream and sent to the heart to be distributed throughout the body. Once used as our fuel, its waste product, carbon dioxide, is then returned through the heart and out the lungs. The heart beats and the body lives. The heart is generating the electrical impulse that runs our nervous system. If we are receiving more oxygen, the body in turn has more energy, more electricity, a stronger heart and lung or cardiovascular system and we are stronger. If the chain is broken in any way, then the whole system becomes depleted and weak. In Yoga we focus on breathing longer and steadier thus increasing the chance of consuming more oxygen i.e.: more energy. We use Pranayama breathing exercises to produce more Prana or energy.

Improved Eating

For me, having the choice of what and how to eat is empowering both for my body and spirit. During my time inhabiting this vessel, I know that my choices will affect my experience and the world around me. I know that what and how I act, including eating, is the footprint that I will be leaving behind. If I can make a simple choice to 'Eat Educated' I can positively affect my body and mind as well as all other living beings and animals. As Yogi Kripalu said, 'May all living beings and animals be happy and healthy." Some philosophers say we have no choice in life. I choose to believe that we do. Choice in how we speak, act and think. Awareness of how what we are doing, saying and living is having an effect on our lives and the lives of those around us in ways we do not understand.

Eating the way, I do now is quite foreign to me. I am still adjusting and sometimes catch myself making food and have to laugh. As a former weight lifter I avoided carbs and fats like the plague. I was all about protein, protein, protein. So I have had a large learning curve. I share with you where Yoga has brought me. It is true, Yoga makes you more mindful, mindful of your thoughts, actions, words and deeds. That mindfulness begins to filter into every aspect of your life, including eating. Slowly over the years I have become more mindful of what is put into our foods by corporations, what is done to the animals that are marketed as our food, how foods are altered and infected with chemicals and how we are ignorant culturally of what is being sold to us as food. I am a firm believer that ignorance is overcome through education and knowing the truth. While I am not a strict vegan, nor am I purist in all things food wise, I know that I can say I am doing the best I can at all time. I feel that I will grow even more from here and evolve as an eater. For now, I am a vegetarian, I try to eat as much living (not cooked above 120 degrees) food as possible, I buy organic and local grown; I call it 'Clean Eating,' little to no processed foods. I don't believe any one way is the right way. I mix in Ayurvedic ideas and principals to modern foods and recipes. There are advantages to all types of eating and disadvantages.

We are all connected. I do what I can to support sustainable methods of living and being. Some ways of commercial agriculture including "Organic" farming can wreak havoc on our top soil and all life surrounding this industry. A vegan diet is a new one in terms of a trend surrounding food. With our furry little friends in mind our vegan friends say no to animal based food including honey. *"I enjoyed pouring my head into the backs of packaging, reading labels at all the health food stores and being a religious vegan. 'Hi, does this have "that" in it and can I get it like this but without that?' I enjoyed all the vegan junk food with the purest intention. Cruelty Free and Karma Free!?? There is no food commercially grown that exists without effecting, killing, and displacing our animal friends. Do you know what a field of wheat looks like after it has been reaped? It is a very bloody harvest. Animals make homes in those fields. Birds nest and feed, gofers, moles, rats, mice, insects, deer, rabbits, turtles, frogs, snakes and spiders. They all live in the fields of these crops. Thousands of animals die and are displaced by commercial agriculture and farming, organic or not. Commercial farms kill to reap our harvest. "*- Trip Waterhouse he recommends reading "Everybody Wants Lunch" by Crazy Owl. So while it may improve your health awareness, stay humble in the journey.

Yoga has been documented in many clinical studies for health and wellbeing benefits. The medical community has begun to use it as an alternative treatment. Many of the ancient Yogi's claims of awareness on the medicinal and health benefits are being proven by modern science. Ultimately, I encourage new or acclaimed students to research and ask questions. Why am I being guided this way and how does this benefit me in this moment. It is individually unique to each person and the variety of personas out there. When I am teaching my Total Engagement Concept I use the instructions to get into the postures and out of them as a guide to focus on the effect of the shapes we are putting our bodies into. I encourage the student to keep their focus on the biological effect of the poses. This is one of the greatest benefits of practicing yoga, fine tuning the minds attention to the processes of the body and mind.

We all often run our bodies on auto pilot. I encourage my students to close their eyes and transition their focus onto their breathing. The breath can be a thread or sutra that ties together the mental faculties and the musculoskeletal with the neurological functions that we all have. Once we switch from autonomic functioning toward consciousness we begin to expand our understanding of the total system we inhabit. If I instruct students to purposefully pause upon hearing the instructions or name of a pose before responding they can become Intune with the awe inspiring functions of their biology. Simplistically speaking, we hear a stimulation, in the case of a yoga class, an instruction or name of posture. Our ear drums translate sound vibration into learned language. This simple feat of hearing and translating is in itself a miracle by most standards. The functioning brain then turns the words into commands. These orders are sent on the bodies delicate yet vastly complex neurological system to the muscular system. Muscles receive their orders and fire or relax to initiate movement. The skeletal system follows the orders and begin to form the shape or pose that the teacher asked for. I call the awareness of the process, slow motion yoga.

The yoga studio is a unique environment not found in most places in life. It is usually a smaller venue, quiet, clean and safe. This feeling of safety allows a student to relax in a way that is rare. Ideally, the yoga studio is filled with compassionate, loving individuals that are supportive and noncompetitive. I have witnessed many friendships formed amongst complete strangers when the studio is cultivated with a sense of community and support. This safe and cocoon like environment called a yoga studio allows the student to be silent and aware whilst forgetting daily demands and stresses. Only then can the student notice the sound and texture of their breathing. This ties the student's attention to a fixed point as opposed to the usual over stimulated and distracted attention. Once that awareness is formed the student can become aware of the subtle processes of the hearing, mental process and how that relates to al functions of the body. I focus my teachings on sound first because it is the most immediate sense. Then I usually move the attention to the more complex of senses, sight, taste (yes even in yoga), feeling, and sent. Once we are in tune with the biodynamics of the body we inhabit, it is quiet enough to ask ourselves why we are here.

Why people practice yoga according to the Yoga Alliance 2006

Give yoga a try and discover what it can do for body and mind.

A central premise in yoga is "everything is connected." That's clear when looking at the health and fitness benefits of yoga that have long been reported by practitioners and are now being confirmed by scientific research.

1. STRESS RELIEF: Yoga reduces the physical effects of stress on the body by encouraging relaxation and lowering the levels of the stress hormone, cortisol. Related benefits include lowering blood pressure and heart rate, improving digestion and boosting the immune system, as well as easing symptoms of conditions such as anxiety, depression, fatigue, asthma and insomnia.

2. PAIN RELIEF: Yoga can ease pain. Studies have demonstrated that practicing Yoga asanas (postures), meditation or a combination of the two, reduced pain for people with conditions such as cancer, multiple sclerosis, auto-immune diseases and hypertension as well as arthritis, back and neck pain and other chronic conditions.

3. BETTER BREATHING: Yoga teaches people to take slower, deeper breaths. This helps to improve lung function and trigger the body's relaxation response.

4. FLEXIBILITY: Yoga helps to improve flexibility and mobility, increasing range of movement and reducing aches and pains.

5. INCREASED STRENGTH: Yoga asanas (postures) use every muscle in the body, helping to increase strength literally from head to toe. Yoga also helps to relieve muscular tension.

6. WEIGHT MANAGEMENT: Yoga (even less vigorous styles) can aid weight control efforts by reducing the cortisol levels, as well as by burning excess calories and reducing stress. Yoga also encourages healthy eating habits and provides a heightened sense of well-being and self-esteem.

7. IMPROVED CIRCULATION: Yoga helps to improve circulation and, as a result of various poses, more efficiently moves oxygenated blood to the body's cells.

8. CARDIOVASCULAR CONDITIONING: Even gentle yoga practice can provide cardiovascular benefits by lowering resting heart rate, increasing endurance and improving oxygen uptake during exercise.

9. BETTER BODY ALIGNMENT: Yoga helps to improve body alignment, resulting in better posture and helping to relieve back, neck, joint and muscle problems.

10. FOCUS ON THE PRESENT: Yoga helps us to focus on the present, to become more aware and to help create mind body health. It opens the way to improved coordination, reaction time and memory.

For more information, please visit www.yogaalliance.org and **www.yogadayusa.org**.

Improved Balancing

One of the most common comments I hear in yoga class especially from new students is that they feel they cannot balance. We either believe we never had balance or we have lost it. What is the best way to improve your balance? Learn easy yoga poses you can do anytime, anywhere using props such as folding chairs, a wall or blocks and straps or better yet a partner. Learning to balance makes you present, centered, and relaxed in difficult situations. Balance also means more than standing on one foot. I often comment during Yoga class that we have the opportunity to create balance in every aspect of our lives. If you exercise hard one day you need to do the opposite to relax and be still in order to balance out the hard exercise you did.

One the way to work at your front door, rather than bending down to put your shoe on, do a one-legged pose and but the shoe on with your knee bent and the foot suspended in front of you. If you worked hard at work all day you need to find time to create stillness and quiet to balance out the hard work you did. If you run you need to sit still, if you cycle or spin you need to lie down and relax, if you have an argument you need to create quiet time. If you go on a spending spree you need to spend some time saving money. Life is all about creating a sense of balance in the physical and all other elements.

I like to offer three ways to improve your physical balance to my classes and private clients. Number one: look to the distance. Look away from you off to the horizon. If you are feeling seasick the instructions are to look at the horizon. If you are relearning how to walk the instructions are to not look down. The same applies for balancing on one foot, look to the horizon and not down at the ground. For where you look you will go. If you look to the horizon you will soar if you look to the floor down, you will go. I always say, the only reason to look down is if money is on the ground.

Number two: your eyes need to relax. If you are distracted by outside sounds, objects moving around then you will focus on the distractions that keep you balancing but if you allow your eyes to go soft focus only on yourself and pointed straight ahead balance will improve. You no longer feel the need to pay attention to distractions and are free to focus only on yourself. Imagine entering a room that is illuminated with bright florescent lighting, the temperature is over one hundred degrees. Now picture the room filled with nearly naked bodies of all types, sweating and moving to the instructions of an also nearly naked teacher. The instructions are barked over a loud speaker and tell you when you can take a sip of water. The room is filled with the strong scent of body odor, mold and wet heat. This is a very popular type of yoga that swept the world. In order to do this a yogic principal must be applied. Pratayahara is the practice of intentionally removing one's senses from being stimulated. Developing the skill of shutting down your input of neurological stimulation from sight, sound, sent, touch and hearing is achievable through deep meditation practices. In a scene like the hot yoga room I was describing, being able to tune out the over stimulation of the room, mostly unpleasant, one is able to make it through the ninety minutes of time that seems like an eternity. This skill takes diligent practice but is vital to improving balance. If a student is in an extremely challenging posture and someone's cell phone rings, the student can tune it out rather than falling out of the posture. I have the challenge of being a deep feeling person. I am easily affected by loud sounds, bright lights, strong smells. Some term it being a highly sensitive person. We are more common than people think, but we are told that we should just relax, or lighten up by others who do not understand. However, we are a specifically skilled type of person. Our strengths are in what we feel. The world to most of us is not so tangible as it is experienced and felt. I get all my information, and intuition from what I am feeling. If I trust that instinct, it never fails to be correct and in my best interest. When I doubt or ignore it, I regret it. Being this type of person and choosing to go to India for three weeks was an enormous challenge for me. India exists to over stimulate in every nook and cranny. My students always ask me what India was like. I can only describe it by saying that there are no words in the English language to describe what India was like. I only survived because I had taken the lesson of withdrawing one's senses literally and studied it intensely in my hot yoga pursuits. When something captures me I usually study the subject to great lengths applying the studies to myself. In India, I delighted in watching the others in my group losing their cool and composure daily. It all added up, the sights, the billions of people in traffic, the smells, bathrooms, and shopping all contributed to someone becoming over stimulated weekly. The only way I made it through each day was by willfully tuning out various stimulations that I had started to notice were becoming overwhelming to me. It was great practice. We are all over stimulated in our nervous system. How can the average student expect to improve their practice every day without proper training? To tune out the constantly stimulating world around is to conserve energy and be focused. It is less of a tuning out and more of an allowing outside stimulation to coexist. I like using outdoor classes as a chance to develop this skill of withdrawal of the senses. We cannot stop the noises or stimulation of sight, sound, taste and hearing. We have to coexist with it all. This practice has been one of my major teachers and helpers. I can be in a crowded and noisy situation and stay balanced. I know enough to leave if it becomes to overstimulating as I am aware of the effects the environment is having on my nervous system. This practice applies to yoga postures in a packed busy studio with cell phones and students falling over as well as in life.

Number three: Breathe and be okay with what is. If you lose your balance breathe and be okay with where you are at now. So often I see people fallout of balance curse or laugh louder than normal and joke about how they can't balance. If we fall out of balance the only solution is to take a deep breath and get back right away without comment or judgement. There are plenty of times later to comment. By attempting to create balance in our lives and our bodies we need to move forward right away, commenting and judgment is a backward energy. If we fall out of balance and focus or create a production about being out of balance, we stay out of balance. If we fall out of balance and breathe and get back into balance without commentary judgement or criticism our balance will return. True in a yoga room and in life. My teacher Swami Kripalu sums it up best by reminding us that the highest spiritual practice is self-observation, without judgement.

Another way of balancing once one has been practicing for a while are inversions. Turning upside down, or lowering your head below your heart can be invigoration and healing. Flowing blood to capillaries that have begun to diminish due to aging. It took me a solid two years of consistent practice, research, study and taking workshops to feel safe doing a headstand without a wall. Head injuries are nothing to take lightly. Placing all your body weight on the tiny and fragile cervical and thoracic spinal connection is not advices for all of us. I am amazed at how much pride and joy a student gets when completing their first headstand. If you take the time to research that part of the spine, which is the nerve super highway and see how jagged the surrounding bone is and how thin the vertebral complex is it would give one pause before expecting it to hold their weight. One fall from a horse, or force of pressure from a fall can stop all body function from the neck down. We take our neck and its importance for granted.

After a neck injury several years ago I was left unable to invert or apply any pressure in my neck. I have tried everything since that day I hit the wrong brake and flew over the handle bars. I remember first the awareness that I was airborne and in a fraction of a second later the distinct smell of my own front teeth burning as I slid across the pavement on my mouth. The emergency room doctor commented later how lucky I was that I wore a helmet. A teenage boy had been in the night before on his shift and having not worn a helmet in the same accident, did not survive. I could have died from this common bike accident. Years of every type of treatment followed, you name it and I have tried it. My neck still hurts every day. The sad thing from me was thinking I might never be able to do Yoga postures again. I had just perfected the free standing head stand the month of my accident.

I attribute my recent return to this anti-aging and mind clearing posture as a result of monthly massages. And learning the proper use of pelvic muscles. Every month I weave a theme into my teachings and spend a month on each theme. After many years of healing from my neck and shoulder injuries, I can return to the theme of head stands and arm balances. It's a good lesson about reaction, fear and what we believe about our abilities. Those crazy looking postures look fun and offer a sense of dramatic accomplishment, but they can be life altering in a negative way if rushed into and poorly performed. I will expand more on this is the chapter Why Not to do Yoga.

I love encouraging others to reach outside their comfort zone. It is only through falling on our head do we learn to get up and try again or quit. I like to observe how others handle this. Some laugh at their foibles others curse and some cry. Me, I jump right in. I need to know the rules of the game or in this case the proper instructions. Then I'm on my way trying it out and learning as much as I can. It's like buzzing down the coast by Big Sur. I can't stand it. Sheer cliffs to ocean on side A, rock and boulders and speeding cars toward us on side B. My travel companion doesn't even seem to notice. However just because I'm praying for my life doesn't mean I don't go. I decided a plan that works for me. I look at the yellow line and let everything else wiz by without a never mind. Then when we get to the destination I enjoy. But I don't let that rough trip or my fear stop me. I go slowly, use caution and proceed with care. Hurting myself has had the benefit of teaching me gentle yoga, yin classes, gaps between breathing, being safe and surviving. In other words, achieving balance. The next time your Yoga Teacher suggest you try turning upside down on the mat observe your reaction. Find a way to manage. Before you know it you'll be flying down that road to success both on and off the mat but safely.

CHAPTER TWO
What is yoga?

In search of the divine we go everywhere. We go to the places of pilgrimage, to sit in temples, follow many paths and disciplines-and ignore our bodies. Your body is the most sacred place of pilgrimage you'll ever come to. It is the dwelling place of the divine spirit; it is the temple of God. Go within and experience the glory of God within you."
-Yogi Amrit Desai

"Everyone has equal claim to yoga and its benefits, but everyone must also observe one primary rule, which is to engage in regular practice. Without practice, even an ordinary task is not accomplished, so how could the extraordinary task of yoga be accomplished? By studying the teachings, a vision of the path may be received, but remember that success does not come in that way. Success comes only through the repeated practice of yoga techniques.:   **-Swami Kripalavanandaji**

Yoga as an Art Form

All martial arts are respected and come from a lineage of teacher or teachings that involve old world respect for the heritage that the art comes from. When entering a center for that martial art, one stops and bows their head to the art and to all the teachers. While Yoga has become 'pop'-ular in the West many have forgotten that it too is an ancient art form that deserves the same emphasis on respect. It is often seen only as an exercise. While Yoga does bring about flexibility, stamina, strength, peace of mind, exercise like movements, breathing exercises and comes served up as hot or acrobatic yoga, it is much more. The true historical significance of the oldest recorded civilization beginning to look at life as something manageable, cannot be rivaled by other, more modern martial arts. With the proliferation of yoga catch phrases and modern marketable gurus have come a lessening of the art of yoga. The word is thrown around as a slogan for the latest problem solving product, mat, clothing line or music festival without its true meaning being known.

A science was created through a specific method of examining, contemplating and studying how life shows up on the planet it all its various forms. This science was first recorded through the Vedic people's practices. This method has been practiced for roughly 5,000 years. Some contemporary voices decry the roots of yoga as debatable, irrelevant, and minor to the health benefits. However, a true scientific approach to results obtained from true practitioners and those that have dedicated their life to the process of yoga has recently been well documented. A consensus throughout the medical world shows that meditation, the first step of yoga, can reverse the effects of injury and illness. Laboratory studies have been held complying with controlled testing regulations to show how meditation and mindfulness change the quality of the minds functions under stress.

Yet many commercialized approaches forget that the art of yoga begins with meditation, contemplation, observations and morals and only uses postures as a small part of the process. In ancient tradition, a student was only accepted to a yoga master after many years of testing and proof that the aspirants aim was pure. A life of denial of pleasure and emotion often accompanied by celibacy was condoned. The student could spend their entire life purifying and never receive the blessing of their teacher while having to watch others achieve spiritual growths without envy or greed. Most times the family would tithe their earnings to the teacher's school or ashram. The son would be bringing the family spiritual karmic blessing by being accepted by the local yoga master as a student. But he would be going against the family norm of an arraigned marriage and other dogmas of society. So it took a bit of a rebellious individual to leave behind the entire family and professional expectations to pursue a spiritual life devoid of material rewards.

Pop Yoga

While many modern voices are earning millions on the huge surge in yoga's popularity few are speaking of the roots, process and scientific approach. If one does not have stellar postures or a sponsor, one is not in the game. Not teaching a festival? Do not have a yoga manager or talent agent? No celebrity endorsements or guest appearances? How many views or posts do you have on your You Tube channel? A fancy sounding Sanskrit word, a new name for a movement, trademarking postures and a hippy look are the markers of a 'good' yogi. Leading teacher trainings and retreats establish you as someone who knows about yoga. Gone are the years of practice, permission and required discipline. A teacher can be made by and out of anyone who has a few thousand dollars and a free weekend.

The modern interpretation of the time proven science of yoga and its complete approach to realization of one's full potential has been dissected and is served in wedges. It is as if just following one part of the formula is as efficient as the whole process. Many are looking to see if there is a shortcut to enlightenment, just as if stretching would answer all mysteries of life. Even those that seem to follow the path correctly stray and fall away as their resolve is tested by fame and speaking engagements. Yoga is being summed up in sound bites and solutions, fashion statements and dollar signs. This is light years away from the beginning of yoga as a deeper understanding of life's greatest mysteries.

What if I told you that you could unlock all the potentialities in your very being? That you possess many gems that you decided to bring to life, to others and to this planet. But that along the way stuff happened to lock it inside you. That stuff is worn like a heavy coat over those gems. We don't even realize that we are wearing a heavy coat and don't understand why our life seems so challenging. Then one day, we wear a hole in the coat and someone points out that they can see a sparkling gem shining through the heavy coat. You can reveal all your hidden gems within through this thing called yoga if you only follow eight steps, or limbs. However, it is useless to try to jump ahead or work the system in reverse. There are literally thousands of well documented case studies dating back thousands of years that prove the process works. The eight steps have been refined, compiled, sourced and examined. When all techniques are followed great things have been proven to happen. Answers are revealed, people's lives transform, their health returns, and the hidden gifts you brought to this world to share come forth.

With all the different information available, it is easy to feel overwhelmed or lost in the variety and information out there. There are only eight steps in the process and a few sub categories to follow in conjunction with one another. The catch is that it is easy to get trapped by one of the categories and just focus on that your whole life. So one must monitor their progress from a removed perspective and observe if they are still engaging in that which no longer serves them. Sometimes teachers and their lessons are right at one stage in one's life, but then one must move on. I understand the plight of 'guru hoppers.' They get bored easily and want the next new solution. It is all so flashy and alluring and 'new.' To find and show off the amazing and beautiful offerings you have to accomplish in this life you must be committed to doing the work of an artisan. Putting in the effort, time and dedication to discipline one's self takes courage and strength.

Standing away from the crowd and looking deeper than the label is only for the brave. Look deeper than this book, or the popular stretching magazine. Ask questions and inquire. Experiment with different approaches. Always ask why? How is this practice benefiting my revealing of the treasures I possess? Am I diving to the calm serene depth or splashing around on the surface because I feel a little better after a 90-minute sweat fest? What is Yoga? The ancients say it takes eight things to do, or eight limbs to practice.

History Says

For me, the Sutras (the threads) are the bible of Yoga. There are many amazing texts and some still to be discovered about Yoga. Most of the Vedic texts have never been written down. Traditions of Yogis throughout the ages have never been translated into English. Even my Guru, Swami Kripalu, has several books I may never get to read because they are not translated. Our current knowledge, is tiny, compared to what has been discovered over thousands of years. That is why Western Yogis who believe they 'know it all' are not practicing Yoga. These Sutras are translated in hundreds of books with varying interpretations and translations. There is a version for every school of thought out there. Find a version you resonate with, an interpretation of these ancient words that seems right to you. For me Satchitananda's reading and insight are the easiest to understand and are filtered to have the lease amount of dogma. The Yoga Sutras of Patañjali have been dated back between 200 B.C. and 200 A.D and remain the primary text of the study of Yoga. Not much is known about Patañjali himself. However, various authorities attribute the compilation of the sutras to Patañjali, who is also referenced as the author of a major treatise on Sanskrit grammar, the Mahabhasya. It may be more like the bible than thought in that it is argued that it may actually have multiple authors. It is assumed that, like the Bible, the Yoga Sutras were constructed by many different authors using the same name. Regardless, the writings provide clear guidelines with exact edicts and ethics for living a Yogic life. It is considered that Patañjali was not the first to write about Yoga - other authors had written before him, and he used their writings in his work. However, as often happens, his text became the authority on the subject. It really approaches Yoga in four parts and treats it as the science it was intended to be. Definition of a Sutra is a stream of consciousness that directs one to manage their mind, body, and self in a systematic Yogic manner. In other words, a sutra provides methods of purifying the mental, physical and emotional bodies in order to bring one into true alignment. One can dedicate their life's work and become a Sutraist, in the pursuit of defining and understanding the Sutras.

The Eight Limbs of Yoga

The yoga sutras translation is loosely accepted as threads, or that which ties together all other aspects of yoga. Without these threads, the whole process is not tied together. Some come to these threads or principles later in their yoga practice, some find them at the first. To help you the most, consider approaching them from where you are on your path, with an open mind and considering heart. When I wanted to really study and learn them from the inside out I used them as my intention in my yoga practice. I would contemplate them daily and watch to see when the subject or in this case intention revealed itself in my daily life. Sometimes they would come up in conversation throughout the day or situations that presented themselves that day. I suggest, if these principals or threads speak to you, begin with one and practice it for a day, a week or as I did, a month at a time. Observe and trust in your own process as you contemplate the one virtue you decided to contemplate. It only takes one and all the rest of them follow. As always, the best place to practice is on oneself.

See if you can apply the principal in your own thoughts, words, actions and deeds throughout your hours, days and months. At first thought, it seems like an easy task to take on, but you will see challenges come to you in this exercise. Notice when your words betray you without even being aware when habits take over. Observe your thoughts as the mind creates them and they rise from awareness into action. See if they comply with the one intention you have set for yourself. Here I have listed some ways to create a working intention from these yoga sutras. Of course I empower you to create your own scientific method to apply these principles in your life. Do your experiment for a minimum of 27 days, but allow a 30-day period in which to experiment. A proper scientific experiment means having a controlled environment, in this case, your mind is your laboratory. Simply observe your thoughts, words, actions and deeds throughout your pre planned time period. Notice when they are in compliance with the principal how your days shows up.

Does practicing the Yama or Niyama (morals and restraints) you have chosen change your interaction with the world as it presents itself. Do your thoughts words actions and deeds fall into alignment or stray far away? Notice how other people speak, think, act and do. Are these participants in your experiment following a different core of observations and actions? Do they feel congruent with your path or rubbing against it? Just notice, keep a record or log, see how it works for a month and move forward. I found after just a month of this experiment, my life was exponentially arriving more in alignment with what I saw for it.

"By firmly grasping the flower of a single virtue, a person can lift the entire garland of Yama and Niyama."
Swami Kripalavanandaji

"Hatha Yoga can be practiced with a primary focus on the external form as a foundation for the spiritual dimensions of the whole body of Ashtanga Yoga. Even when the physical discipline is practiced alone, it can be impregnated with intention to plant the seeds of the mental and spiritual dimensions that expand Hatha Yoga from an exclusively physical discipline into a psychosomatic and bio spiritual discipline." **Yogi Amrit Desai and the Yoga Sutras**

Yoga Sutras 2.29 Yama-Niyama-asana-pranayama-Pratyahara-dharna-dhyana-samadhyayo astavangani

Yama: Strong willpower for restraint

Niyama: Strong willpower for observance and application of truth

Asana: Physical and mental exercise including postures.

Pranayama: Transformation of individual energy, physiological and psychological, into cosmic energy.

Pratyahara: Displacement and sublimation of psychic energy

Dharana: Fixation of mind on various places, internal or external

Dhyana: Sublimation of mind into Being

Samadhi: Evolution of consciousness from individuality to universality.

Patañjali who is the credited author of the Yoga Sutras has controversy surrounding his authorship or even existence. He laid out the systematic path called ashtanga, which literally means eight limbs. There are eight ideas to guide a student towards a productive and successful life. Some call them the commandments of yoga. I like to say they are the encouragements of yoga, not commands and they come without self-repudiation or guilt.

Yama is sometimes misconstrued as karma, which is open to interpretation and discussion. I always advice with any new concept to the student that the practice must begin inwardly. Trying to practice these outwardly and on others can be frustrating and unfulfilling. If we try applying these ideas or principals on our own thoughts words action and deeds first, we can become aware of how we are treating ourselves. Once we improve our personal relationships with our self-identity, then we can begin to work outwardly. If these ideas, or any uplifting ideas take root inside first, they easily translate to others.

Yamas are: 1. Ahimsa: non-violence 2. Satya: truthfulness 3. Asteya: non-stealing 4. Brahmacharya: continence 5. Aparigraha: non-covetousness, non-hoarding.

Niyamas are best practiced through watching one's actions as they move on their path of life. My teacher likes to say be the witness not the judge and jury. Watch how you interact with the world as it presents itself to you. Become aware of the choices you are making in life.

The five niyamas are: 1. Saucha: cleanliness 2. Samtosa: contentment 3. Tapas: heat; spiritual austerities, self-discipline 4. Svadhyaya: study of the sacred scriptures and of one's self 5. Isvara pranidhana: surrender to a higher power.

Way of Life

Yoga is more than knowing postures and speaking poetic terms. It becomes a way of life. The more you live your Yoga the more you will naturally embody the principals. Yoga is not something we do; it is something we are. Using the guideposts of Yoga, Yama and Niyama, as your personal ethics and morals, will keep you in a sacred space. By referring to these guide posts, you can check in and see if your actions, thoughts, words and deeds are in alignment with your principles. Look at yourself and see if you are following the path of light that you have chosen to be a part of. Are your interactions with others putting you in the space of trust and non-harming? If you feel compromised by something that someone is saying or actions they are taking, ask yourself if this is stemming from anything you may have said or done. If it is not, then distance yourself from that person politely.   If you feel that because of temptation or just the natural part of being human, you have taken a choice that has led you to an area where your ethics and morals are in question, try not to judge yourself. Take the actions needed to bring yourself back to center. Admit that you have strayed off your true path and realign yourself.   The more we create a safe environment to have a life transformative experience, the less we will succumb to momentary fascination.

CHAPTER THREE
Styles of Yoga

"While honoring all yoga traditions, Amrit Yoga expands the popular concept of yoga as a physical discipline into bio-spiritual dimensions. It creates new possibilities for widening the range of healing modalities and self-discovery. The concepts are adaptable to various levels of healing and therapeutic applications, as well as for spiritual growth."

-Yogi Amrit Desai

"The body benefits most when the postures are performed with a full understanding of their purpose and intended effects. Avoid straining the body through over-enthusiastic practice. Perform postures only within the limits of your strength, stopping when you feel tired. Begin by performing and holding easier postures with conscious breathing. Work gradually to accomplish more difficult postures, and avoid forcing the body into them prematurely. After achieving a difficult posture, increase your endurance by systematically lengthening your holding time. Work to your own limit, and do not judge your progress by the progress of another. Follow this guidance. Otherwise, the body can be harmed."

-Swami Kriaplanandaji

The design of this great system of eight limbs of yoga is to serve the evolution of all mankind. Inherent in the foundation tracing back thousands of years is the idea of maximizing one's human experience on all planes of existence. To reduce suffering and separation and create unity and oneness is the definition of the word

Yoga, Yog, to Yoke or draw out your maximum potential. How can you create unity when you are in an uncomfortable situation, in stress without knowing why you are there?

If you are new to Yoga, experienced or just checking it out to see if you want to do it, why is the beginning. Each posture should be for a purpose, a reason, physical, mental, energetic, psychic, emotional, and awareness. Yoga classes should, be intelligent, well thought through, serve the needs of the students and be presented in an easy to understand, educated and noncompetitive manner. They should not be dangerous, thrown together or made up on the spot with no direction

Before picking the class you want to take tell me what your why is? No really, what is it you want from what you are doing? Why is the class asking you to do a specific something and what are you getting out of it? I ask this several times in class as a leader. Mostly I get blank stares. How can we know what we want if we don't know who we are or what we truly hope to get out of something? Have you ever felt blindly led into a situation without knowing why you are there and then left with a feeling of being lost? This does not just apply to Yoga, we all do it all the time. Whether you never pick up a Yoga mat or try a class, you can use these guide posts I have created to determine exactly what it is you want and how to get it now. If you are considering Yoga or currently practicing, this self-exploration can create instant clarity for you on your path.

I remember when I first went to my teachers institute in Florida and was introduced to a Kirtan. This form of music is often played before a meeting with the teacher. Coming from exercise yoga, this was my first authentic experience. The words were all sung in Hindi or Sanskrit. Musicians were playing the drums and various instruments from India I had never seen nor heard. Everyone was singing or swaying along to the songs. Some were in deep states of trance. I was out of my element. I remembered my mother's advice when I first moved to California, to watch out for cults. For a boy from Kansas, this setting certainly fit the bill. My life has led me on one unexpected adventure after another. I have seen all types of cities, states, countries and people. I have dined with the super-rich, washed dishes and flipped burgers along-side worker bees, traveled Europe and Japan and sat in the dirt in India and Bali, but I will always be a little boy from Kansas. I was out of my element my first time seeing and hearing this music as we waited for the teacher. I could only stay in the room for one song before leaving due to my fear that my brain was being sucked out. It was too new and foreign to me, these songs and everyone signing together. I had the same feeling the first time I heard Kumbaya around the campfire in Boy Scouts.

It was so new to me and I was so uneducated about the idea of Kirtan I could not sit in the room. I was sitting alone, wondering what I had got myself into on my quest to find out about authentic yoga and wanting to run back to the safety of the gym yoga I knew, when the Guru's daughter, Kamini Desai, approached me. This is a woman in the true definition. I know she likes to be treated as one of the crowd and I have grown to know people that can pal around with her. However, to me, she carries herself and appears to me as if one of the Goddesses from India embodied and walked out of a temple. She has the energy and presence, to me, of my Guru, a great teacher, yet the femininity of mythological proportions. She seems at once, ethereal yet very much of the body. One time she gave me a ride to the airport which was an hour and half in the car and I was literally paralyzed with awe by her beauty and energy into a state of very rare, for me, silence. I really worked hard on clarifying to myself that I did not feel this way because she was the Guru's daughter, some sort of star. I made sure I saw her as independent of him and looked at her as her own person. It was her own untapped energy I was feeling. I knew that even she was not aware of her potential power and strength and the liquid energy she transmitted or if she was, she did not wield it. I also felt the presence of a male teacher who stands over her left shoulder and the feeling of her mother, also a strong woman, who stands beside her right side. I have always been empathic and felt deeply. My intuition is feeling based. To me she feels like liquid amber, infused with all the power of masculine and feminine. I so wanted to speak, but at the time, I was entranced.

As she sat across from me outside the Kirtan, she asked if I was ok. I explained to her, in some fumbled way, that I was new to all this yoga business and had only done work out yoga up to that point. I was frightened and uncomfortable by the music and trance like state everyone in the other room was in. I wanted to know what yoga meant to them. I was overwhelmed and intimidated by the deeper meaning, having no understanding of the reasons for the foreign and seemingly religious sounds. Everyone seemed happy and content and were participating so it must be for a reason. I was confused and felt lost. I did not know why I was at the institute after all and I wanted to know if I had to become a Hindu to practice deeper yoga. I told her I was raised somewhat loosely as a Christian, studied Buddhism, Native American beliefs and meditated but if I had to become Hindu then I should probably leave because all the gods and goddesses frightened me. I had lost my 'Why', why I was there.

As she lovingly listened, I could see a glowing light inside the iris of her eyes. A light of empathy, compassion, understanding and deep knowledge. I felt she had been here before with someone else having this same conversation yet she projected a depth of love that embraced me. It was a rare feeling for me to be so completely understood and supported without judgement. She explained to me that she understood, and with the slightest smile reassured me that no one was wanting me to become a Hindu. She suggested that I not even concern myself with the words but if it felt right to me, to try to feel the sound vibration the music was creating. That the vibration of sound can be very powerful and used as a healing tool. Now she was speaking my language, feeling something. If I could allow myself, when it was right for me, to just sit in the room and see what I felt I might have a different perspective. She let me know that the musicians sing songs from all faiths and that it had nothing to do with religion but was a form of meditation or prayer. I felt instantly at ease. I can't say I ran back into the room and became a lover of yoga song, but I felt comforted. I felt safe. I was starting to understand what yoga was about, unity, merging, vibration, energy, not words and dogma or postures and competition, but the place where we all meet. I felt safe.

This feeling unlocked a lot of understanding for me in that second. It was as if her presence created a quickening of understanding in me. I based my whole future of yoga and teaching in that moment. If I can, as a teacher create a safe and loving, non-judgmental environment for my students, they can feel comfortable enough to release fear and gain experience which leads to understanding. I know how confusing it can be to walk into yoga at the beginning. Not knowing what it all means. How does one start out, what does it all mean, why is everyone else doing it when it seems so foreign at first? If you can discover your Why, why you are checking out this yoga thing, you will be able to approach it without fear.

Find Your Why?

According to the Amrit Yoga Institute

INTENTION INVITES INTEGRATION Intention is the "why" and 'how" of Amrit Yoga-practice. Intention is what keeps you motivated to stay in "witness", to purify the body and continue moving towards integrating the separative parts of self. It is through intention that the soul recognizes its destiny, the understanding, the "aha" that begins to make sense out of a senseless world. The overall intention or "ultimate" intention sets the stage for which all the discipline and commitment of your practice is oriented. Whatever your intention, it is that idea that will return you to " center " when engaged in daily activities, relationships or the workplace.

Supporting or "working" intentions are used to remove subconscious issues, 'karmic patterns, ingrained beliefs and attitudes in an unpurified blocked body that may make the "ultimate" intention impossible to identify or too esoteric to relate to. Supporting intentions are short-term intentions that are used in conjunction with your ultimate intention. The working intention must always be aimed at supporting the ultimate intention.

An example of an ultimate intention is peace. Say you are constantly in conflict with yourself over body image and bring to mind a working intention of a beautiful body to attract a male. You could end up with a diet producing a beautiful body but maintaining it may not bring you continued peace. Whereas a working intention "of a healthy body to support my practice of yoga and pursuit of my highest intention of peace", may bring you just that.

In the case of the ultimate intention of surrender, this can be a bit lofty to practice in the daily world. Whenever you find yourself in conflict, an irritating relationship or self-depreciation, the question that arises is, "am I allowing what is to be?" And with a gentle nudge, you edge yourself back to center, back to the direction you want to experience life and how you want to present yourself living that life. Intention defines your practice of Amrit Yoga and ultimately your way of living life. It produces guidance and structure for every step of the way towards integration.

Differing Schools of Yoga (a partial list)

Yoga schools at a glance

- **Ananda:** Developed by Swami Kriyananda, a direct disciple of Paramhansa Yogananda. The emphasis is on self-realization.

- **Anusara:** As taught by John Friend, this school focuses on flowing with grace and is based on principles and spirals of alignment.

- **Ashtanga:** Developed by K. Pattabhi Jois, this yoga gives you a serious athletic workout.

- **Baptiste Method of Yoga:** Developed by Magaña and Walt Baptiste, this school is based on Raja yoga; the focus is on mind and meditation.

- **Baptiste Power of Yoga:** Developed by Sherri Baptiste, this school brings together flowing postures, breathing techniques, and yoga philosophy.

- **Bikram:** Developed by Bikram Choudhury, this school presents a series of 26 static holding postures practiced in a room heated to 110° Fahrenheit.

- **Himalayan Institute:** Developed by Swami Rama from a lineage of sages of the ancient cave monasteries of the Himalayas, the focus is on meditation.

- **Integral:** Swami Satchidananda's Integral yoga is a major component of Dr. Dean Ornish's groundbreaking work on reversing heart disease.

- **Iyengar:** Developed by B.K.S. Iyengar, this school emphasizes attention to detail and the precise alignment of postures.

- **Kripalu:** This school puts great emphasis on proper breathing, alignment, and the coordination of breath and movement.

- **Kundalini:** Developed by Yogi Bhajan, this school emphasizes classic poses, breathing, the coordination of breath and movement, and meditation.

- **Paramahansa Yogananda:** This is the Kriya yoga self-realization fellowship; the emphasis is on the spiritual and on meditation.

- **Power Vinyasa Yoga:** Developed by Baron Baptiste, this is a sweat-based, synchronized, dynamic-flow yoga practiced in a room heated to 85–90°F.
- **Sivananda:** This school follows a set structure that includes pranayama, classic asanas, and relaxation.
- **Viniyoga:** Developed by Sri T. Krishnamacharya and carried on by his son, T.K.V. Desikachar, this school is a methodology for developing practices for individual conditions and purposes.
- **Vivekananda:** This school offers a spiritual brand of yoga.

The amount of styles of Yoga can be slightly overwhelming at first glance. The only way to know which version of this ancient art that has been adapted to the demands of the modern world is to first know why one wants to do yoga. Usually the why is not the first answer we give ourselves. Many people try styles based on what their friends are doing, or a recent article they may have read and liked, a fashion trend or a new diet goal. As you read this ask yourself how those new year's resolutions have been working out for you? Most of us drop those resolutions in the first ninety days from their making. Take the time and inward focus to sort out the ego's goals from true needs and desires. We need food, shelter, sex and happiness to survive. When we boil down our motivators, they are usually based on these principals at first. Setting those aside, we can begin to explore the real needs for our evolution beyond the primal wants. Once we move beyond our first instinctual drives we can begin to look at a higher purpose for our actions, even the ones that drive us to try yoga. Taking the time to find out why we are being drawn to a particular style or teacher we can find the right one for our needs.

CHAPTER FOUR
What's my type of class?

Make the time to take as many different styles of Yoga that call out to you. Don't just get locked into one style and think that is Yoga. Yoga is indefinable. It, to me, is a martial art, and a discipline. It takes fortitude, practice, experience and passion. There are so many styles of 'Yoga' being invented every year here in America. You could go your whole life learning. What I think you will find, is one style will be 'Your Style' for a while, maybe months, maybe years, then you will evolve into something else. This way you are climbing a ladder of Yoga.

I don't think it is beneficial to 'Guru Hop' where you take one class from this person and that. I think it is good to see if a style calls to you and then get absorbed in it as much as you can. When it no longer satisfies see what the next progression would be. My Guru has a saying; "Yoga is popular, what is popular is NOT Yoga". I see this in all the trends and 'new' ways of doing Yoga. While it is fantastic that Yoga is exploding in our culture where it is much needed, one should ask, why they are doing Yoga. What is the perceived result desired from this form or practice? Is standing on my head on an unstable board in the ocean really going to benefit my journey? What is the reason you are on your Yoga path? Why are you there?

If the teacher, style, presentation of information, lifestyle, morals, ethics, heck, even the music are not serving your higher good, why endure? As my first meditation teacher says in her book 'Meditations for Miracles', "The only virtue in suffering is realizing that you do not need to suffer". I do not relate to boot camp style training or the drill sergeant you must be in pain to gain mentality. I do believe in discipline but that is an entirely different lesson than being demeaned and in pain. If you are taking a style of Yoga or what is being called Yoga, ask yourself how it is serving you and your greatest good.

Sample Class Types

Different Class Formats (these are generic descriptions found at most studios.)

Traditional Yoga. Amrit Method. Level I. Medium Intensity.	Intro to Amrit Method Level 1	Passed down from teachers from India, Amrit Yoga is a metaphor for life. The skills of mindful attention and meditative awareness you develop on the yoga mat extend to challenges you encounter in life. Painful transition periods, relationships and crises can become opportunities and openings for personal transformation.
Kundalini Yoga	Yoga of Energy	A Traditional Yoga posture class. Learn the art of authentic Yoga with breath, stretching, postures and exercises ending with mindfulness exercises. Have a transformation, stimulates the major glands in your body for healing, change old habits into new. Learn how to balance your energy centers, control the waves of the mind with scientific techniques. Royal ancient yoga in its purest form. Authentic, unchanged, the real deal.

Yoga Nidra, Amrit Method. Low Intensity.	Guided Meditation	Non Spiritual approach to learning how to incorporate stress reduction and focus into your life. Learn the basics of mental games that create meditation techniques. Enhance your life, relax, let go and destress. From breathing techniques, to postures that help with insomnia to getting the mind too quiet. Bring a blanket and eye pillow and prepare to let go.
Children's Yoga	Level One	Moms or Dads bring the little one and prepare to start laughing and having fun while doing yoga, the little ones teach us to have a sense of humor, go with the flow, to stay present and to embrace change. The connection between the parent and child is deepened through the principles of Yoga.
Gentle Yoga Low intensity.	Restorative	Consists of easy movements, long stretches and deep breathing, meant to calm and revitalize. This class is appropriate for students of every ability, age, and fitness level. Each class ends with a new stress reduction technique.
Stretching Low Intensity	Restorative	Stretch, plain and simple, for all people who want to stretch tight areas. A class for the non-Yogi looking to find a way to move slowly through stretching and core strengthening exercises. Start with a held

		flexibility position. Perfect for those over 60.
Mat Pilates Med. to High Intensity	Pilates	Pilates primarily aims to work the core muscles. This includes the stomach and lower back, as well as the pelvic muscles, buttocks, thighs and spine. By working on the core, you can attain better posture, breathe easier and better, improve your balance, control the flow of air and blood within the body and improve your concentration. Core Pilates exercises do not consist of traditional abdominal work with a lot of repetition. Instead, they are more akin to yoga, where you hold a single pose or movement throughout its full range.
Weights & Yoga Med to High	Yoga with Weight: Sculpt	Do a Yoga posture, then ad in weights to fire it up. Strengthen muscle, stretch and increase flexibility, leave feeling strong not sore. Light to medium weights. Travel from warm up, through core exercises, to balancing and a Vinyasa flow all with and without weights
Yoga Basics Low Intensity	Level One	Postures for every level from beginner to advanced. Start with this introduction to Yoga, level One and progress to Salute Two. Spend more time on the basic moves; understand how to do them properly avoiding injury as your progress. Ask

		questions, break down of postures, understand more
Hatha Yoga Low to Med Intensity Level I	Level One	A combination of holding and flowing. The most common style of yoga taught in the west. Should combine some more challenging poses or sequences followed by cooling postures. Sun and Moon.
Power Yoga. Med. to High Intensity Level II	Power Yoga Level Two	Constantly moving with a strong core section. A dynamic flow of powerful asanas synchronized with breathing techniques used to generate internal body heat. This, combined with two important internal 'bandhas' (body locks), induces profuse sweating during the sequence, which eliminates toxins. There is a dramatic increase in energy and well-being. This system is not for beginners. Ashtanga based.
Yoga Flow Med to High Intensity and Cardio.	Yoga Flow	Yoga Flow is the perfect blend of core work, Yoga, sports stretch, dance stretch, and athletics that will help you burn calories and build muscle! It's about way more than just flexibility. The dynamic blend of movement increases strength, balance, and agility, while being a good workout It does not usually provide a mind/body experience.

Say No

When choosing your teacher and class, I empower you to say no to your teacher, or style of class when being asked to do something that does not make any sense or feel right to your anatomy. I am not encouraging insubordination where you say no to anything that makes you feel uncomfortable. I have had that student in class and it is very disruptive. I encourage you to ask why the teacher is asking you do to do a posture or shape and if it does not resonate with you, find a modification that does, within the context of the class. I do want you to ask why the teacher is asking you to do something if it does not make any sense. I remember once in teacher training the lead teachers were showing us a modification to a posture that I was not sure was safe or what was the benefit in doing the modification. I was pretty sure the root posture, thread the needle, was not even a yoga posture. But the modification seemed especially risky as it involved a twist with the main contact point potentially being the cervical spine. My neck wanted further explanations. I remember raising my hand and trying to politely ask why this modification was being taught and its benefits. The teachers looked at each other and everyone was quiet as they had just been absorbed in learning how to do something 'new' and 'fun'. No one had thought to ask why. The answer I got was that it was a way to add a backbend to the posture. Not good enough for me. I wanted to know how to teach this if I decided to teach it, in the safest way possible without anyone risking paralysis because they fell over on their neck. Not in my class.

Some teachers are taught to teach similar postures or instructions that make no sense to me, or that seem harmless until it is put in the practical application of a real class with real students.

That is why in my teacher trainings the teachers to be are put immediately in the class room with real students and not sequestered in a class room for weeks before encountering a real student. Friends and family are too complimentary and not challenging enough. One very common instruction given to new teachers to be is to begin your classes in child's posture. Upon further application and contemplation, I do not subscribe to this practice in my classes. I encourage you as a student to be this thoughtful and examine why you're being asked to do anything that seems rote or routine without explanation. Ask why if it makes no sense and if an intelligent, practical answer cannot be given, skip it. Put Thought into Postures: Don't start with child's pose (Balasana or Garbasana). Child's Pose is a popular posture for teachers to start their class in. Below I state reasons that you should not practice child's posture unless you're warmed up and in great health. I never start in this posture and find it very unwise for most students to begin here. My main concern is safety first for my students. A teacher should create a safe environment for a student's own growth. A teacher should know exactly why they are teaching postures to their students. When considering the benefits of a Yoga pose, the question should be asked, why not do a posture? I've found in twelve years of teaching all body types that the majority of students are ill equipped for this pose, myself included.

Instructions for Garbasana (Child's Pose): Kneel on the floor. Touch your big toes together and sit on your heels, then separate your knees about as wide as your hips or as wide as your mat. Exhale and lay your torso down between your thighs. Lay your hands on the floor alongside your torso, palms up, and release the fronts of your shoulders toward the floor. Or extend your arms out shoulders width with palms down.

Purported Benefits Gently stretches the hips, thighs, and ankles. Calms the brain and helps relieve stress and fatigue. Most of the population has tight ankles from wearing shoes and not stretching. This position hyper-flexes stiff ankle joints and connective tissue. Ever twist your ankle? This is essentially what you're doing to the top of your foot with your body weight pressing on delicate bone. Tight knees and injuries to the knee joint can cause a myriad of issues for the many people. Shin splints, runners knee, Achilles tendinitis, floating knee-cap, swelling around and behind the knee are just a few of the external issues that can be compounded by the pressure in this pose, especially on a cold joint. Internally, the potential of a twist in the joint leading to a meniscus tear is enough warning in this position to warrant not being here cold (without warming up). A meniscus surgery can potentially require a cadaver transplant.

We haven't even made it to the hips yet. The potential external rotation of the hips with the added body weight pressure can cause an inflammation of bursitis and sciatica. The compression of the femoral artery and contraction of the hip flexor can cause numbness and loss of blood flow throughout the legs. Most of the population have tight hamstrings and this posture creates a sustained hamstring contraction making things tighter.

The extended arm version can create a contraction of tight neck and shoulder muscles aggravating the upper body. Rotator cuff injuries are common in most individuals. In this posture we are irritating tight shoulders and potentially adding stress to the delicate rotator cuff tendons and tissue. To compensate, most students will lock out their elbows. Tendinitis is another common ailment. Even with the hands back by the feet version of this pose there is a rotation in the forearm to turn the palms up which is a major irritant of tendinitis.

This posture can cause a bowing of the back due to tight back muscles. This pulling can culminate in the sacral and lumbar area. Never allow someone to push or try to straighten out your back in this position especially if you're not warmed up. I find most students place pressure on their forehead causing compression in the back of their neck, another common site of injury. As a neck injury survivor, I find this pose unbearable even with my chin tucked in. Another supposed benefit is stress reduction. However, when we have pressure in our chest and abdomen it can be difficult to breath. This posture puts most students in an abdominal contraction with rounded shoulders and tightened ribs, making it challenging to take a deep or prolonged breath. Yoga should start with a deep centering breath technique not available with a compressed abdomen. For a student suffering from panic attacks or claustrophobia this is a frightening posture to begin with.

I will skip the contraindications for pregnancy. Suffice it to say this posture is good for children. An average individual, new to Yoga or not, may find this posture uncomfortable and potentially damaging; especially when it is the first shape they are asked to assume with a cold, tight and stiff body. All the top ten sports injuries can be aggravated by this 'restful' posture. For these reasons and more I will never start my Yoga classes from here. I'd rather have you facing me so I can see your smile as you sit upright and breathe deeply with me. I share this with you in hopes that you will see how much contemplation is meant to be placed on each element of yoga. Even the most basic of poses are meant for our deepest contemplations. In some traditions, months or even years are spent on one posture before the student can progress.

Personal Choice

Ultimately when seeking out the right class for you, keep in mind that it is deeply personal to you and what your body needs at that time. After hurting my neck in Scotland, my body needed to take healing yoga and restorative classes. These were unfamiliar territory to me. I did nothing slow before the injury, but I was in so much pain that I had to find an alternative or give up my practice. The thought of never doing yoga again brought tears to my eyes. I knew I had to find a different type of class than the physically rigorous postures I had been doing. I had just perfected my headstand the same month I went over the handle bars and had been deep into hot yoga which, although not by design, but by environs is highly competitive. I really did not want to give up my pursuit of my posture holy grail, the Scorpion. In this posture the student is balanced on forearms with the feet on the head and the body suspended above them like the tail of a scorpion. It is a daunting looking pose. But I was close!

Now with sever whip lash that I will be dealing with the rest of my life, I had to go back to the drawing board and seek out a different type of class. I researched all types of healing yoga, yoga therapy, Yin yoga, gentle yoga, restorative yoga and all kinds of hippy sounding derivatives. I remember the first gentle class being like a personal hell. It reminded me of my first hot yoga class in the Key West. It took all I had not to run out of the room. The teacher had her, what I call, 'rainbows and unicorns' voice. It was so saccharine sweet and full of poetic quotes and analogies that involved floating and flying on puffy clouds into clear blue skies. All I could think about was that this would be the yoga teacher if they had one in 'One Flew Over the Cuckoo's Nest.' Most of the class was done rolling around on the floor and involved prolonged holding. I was used to moving and flowing in Hatha classes or tortured holding in hot yoga. I knew this teacher was not the right one for me, but unfortunately, my body responded very well to the stretches. It was as if my body was craving being cradled.

Having the injury forced me to look at a type of yoga, mostly occupied by an older crowd and geared toward healing or recovering from injuries or life's bumps in the road. The students were supportive and friendly. Try to get someone in the hot yoga world to hang out after class and engage in conversation. It generally speaking, does not happen. These gentle yoga people seemed like they really cared, like the teachers. This ultimately led me to design my yoga studio around the principals of safety and caring. Looking at these restorative classes taught me to slow down in life and yoga. It was exactly what I needed at that time as I journeyed into the deeper practice of my Guru's style of yoga. I began to learn to teach and use props such as blocks, straps, and chairs to assist in postures unreachable to a lot of students. This led me to taking Iyengar classes and learning about that lineage. I met many amazing teachers in Iyengar that were very firm and disciplined and wore clothes that covered their body, unlike the exercise and hot yoga world I had been in up to that point. This led me to John Friend and his workshops which took students on long journeys from a very basic pose into the most complex without the student knowing where they were headed. It always surprised me at the end of one of John's classes or workshops where we ended up because the journey was so subtle. I admit, I was very resistant to this type of long holding in one posture and really challenged by the seemingly artifice voice many gentle teachers adopt. It sounds to me like they are talking to puppies and kittens. Because of that though, I added a whole section in my 200 hour TEC Yoga training program that focuses on developing an authentic speaking voice drawing on my many years of public speaking and theatre training.

Ultimately, my neck injury forced me to investigate all types of classes that normally I would have avoided like the plague. This reinforced the importance of being open to investigating all types of yoga and classes outside my safety box. I encourage all students to do the same. Make sure you're in the right class. Is the teacher well prepared? Have they spent time developing a specific sequence around an intention? Or is the class a hodgepodge of their favorite postures not in the best interest of the student? When trying new classes ask yourself if the resistance you are experiencing is because it is truly the class you need? Once a style of class resonates with you, go deep into it. Try all the teachers in your area or online that are teaching in that style. Stick to that format of class until the body tells you it is ready to try a different class. Make sure the teacher is keeping you safe. I always tell my student that I am just their yoga life guard, keeping them safe. The main focus is the class style and theme and how it is serving the students. As always, ask why you are there in that class and what is it doing for you.

CHAPTER FIVE
Who is the right teacher?

"There is a magnet in your heart that will attract true friends. That magnet is unselfishness, thinking of others first; when you learn to live for others, they will live for you."

— Paramahansa Yogananda

"Two are better than one, because they have a good return for their toil. For if they fall, one will lift up his fellow; but woe to him who is alone when he falls and has not another to lift him up. Again, if two lie together, they are warm; but how can one be warm alone? And though a man might prevail against one who is alone, two will withstand him."

-Ecclesiastes 4:9-12

There are many different ways to teach. However, I do not believe in reinventing the wheel. There is an entire industry of professional teachers of all types in the world. There is a whole cottage industry on how to effectively teach others. There are elementary school teachers with their own unique techniques of dealing with children learners. Motivational speakers have their own language and methods of teaching that are unique to their profession. University professors have at some point looked into the way people learn and how to teach different types of learners. Any teacher worthy of the title teacher has at some point self-taught themselves or been trained in how to effectively distribute that which they are meaning to communicate, and, this is the important part, make sure that it is received and understood by the student. This is a skill and talent and that which makes the excellent teachers stand out as leaders and life transformers.

One of my favorite teacher trainings I led had a student who had also been a teacher. She helped me see the importance of researching and learning more effective ways of teaching others. She shared with me the techniques and tools she had learned at University. I have always found the subject of communication fascinating. Having worked in the broadcast industry for so many years, I knew the important of making a simple statement that communicated effectively the point one was trying to make. I am not talking about debate, which is its own, stand alone, form of discussion. That is a different conversation. In the broadcast world, you need to get things out in sound bites that either sum up the story using the highlights or points of interest, or try to capture the importance of the message in a sentence that gets the listener intrigued to hear more about the subject. Being a shy introverted child and young adult, but knowing I wanted to be more gregarious, I took many communication classes. I enrolled in theatre, public speaking, voice over classes and worked through my shyness and feelings of not being heard.

Communication is like throwing a ball. You want to send a communication, equivalent to tossing a ball to a friend. The other person has to receive it in order to throw it back. It is important that the receiver understands the communication and acknowledges it before tossing the ball back. By giving a successful acknowledgment, it can dissolve any misunderstandings. Person A sends a communication to Person B across time and space. Person B receives the communication and needs to give a strong acknowledgement. This acknowledgement is needed by Person B but more importantly by Person A- the communicator. If an acknowledgement is not audibly received, the communicator has no way of knowing if the message has been received and accepted. If the message was not clear, Person B- the receiver can ask for more information. This communication continues until both Persons A and B feel they understood the communication. True communication can handle and resolve any problem in the universe.

This is the way the world has always communicated since the invention of writing letters. A person would send their communication to another person. The other person would have time to contemplate what they found in the letter before responding. They would write back based on what was in the original letter. Stating that they understood or asking further questions. If no letter was ever received back, the original sender would not know if their letter had made it to the correct person. We seem to only do this in today's world with fax machines. We wait for a confirmation that the fax was received before moving on. If we do not get the confirmation, we assume it did not go through and we resend. However, with email and texting we often just assume the other person has received it. You can hear it all the time, people say that they did not receive the email or text and blame it on the technology if they had not wanted to receive the communication. In some instances, it is actually never received, but it makes a perfect excuse for not hearing or receiving communication.

When you are choosing your teacher I would advise you to observe. Are they an effective communicator? See if your teacher is skilled in teaching a variety of different learning types. Notice if what they are trying to communicate is acknowledged by the students in the class. Watch and see if your teacher makes sure they are heard and understood. Or do they just barrel through with their agenda? Will your teacher adapt to unexpected student limitations or challenges, or get annoyed at any questions or delays? I have found that as an attendee of yoga teacher trainings, not much time is spent on learning the fine art of teaching others how to teach. Most yoga teacher's schooling was spent on how to do a posture and the proper bodily alignment. Not much time was invested on making sure that they are understood by a diverse group of students. Look at your life, do you have a favorite teacher, Ted Talk, You Tube channel? How do your favorite teachers communicate that makes them resonate with you? Look for that quality in your yoga teacher.

You want to hear the teacher, ensure that you are doing things correctly avoiding injury and being heard if you have a question or concern. One of the greatest teaching tools that I have learned from is listening and observing my teacher giving public talks and how he patiently waits to hear the students question. He usually responds with questions of his own that are like a laser cutting to the source of the question. He guides and directs the student to their own self-discovery and the student often comes up with the answer their selves. This empowers the student and creates the sense of teamwork. It dismantles the paradigm that the teacher is something of an anomaly that must know something special that only they know. Because of watching my teacher, I teach from complete place of humility and service. I have no patience for being talked down to or demeaned in any way which is a very easy role for a teacher to slip into. I try to always come from a place of equal team work in communicating. See if you feel this way after your yoga class.

The Voice

The voice is a great place to start. It is my way of reading a person's demeanor. Having spent so much time and energy researching the voice and how it is used as an effective means of communication, it is the very first observation I make as a student and as a communicator. Vocal training, public speaking, projection for the actor, diction and voice over classes many has enhanced my ability to use my voice as an effective means of communication. I can easily modulate my tonality and volume to affect a mood or meaning in my directions as a teacher. On many occasions I have experienced or had others comment that some teacher's voices were challenging to listen to for an hour. They felt the teacher's voice was too high pitched, nasally, soft and low in volume or just not efficient. Good teachers should want to support the student by creating a safe zone for them. What if, just by your voice, you could make someone 'feel' what you were trying to relay. This is the basis of Sanskrit, the ancient language of Yoga. It is an energy exchange. Funny enough it is also the premise of the motion picture 'Dune'. As actors in theatre we can relay to the audience the mood of our character. Just because the character I am playing is angry, I do not need to go through the stress of actually getting angry. It helps to back up your voice with an emotion on stage but in a yoga class, the emotion can also be conveyed with the use of the voice. I have developed a powerful vocal tone that I have to be cautious to modulate and control in an enclosed environment like a class room. Often times 'the Voice' comes out by accident in its full emotions when I do not intend it to. People usually take it personally and I have learned to immediately catch it and explain that I did not mean to sound so powerful in that moment. The tone of voice shows our concern for the audience and determines in the minds of the audience whether or not we are sincere. The audience may say a speaker is boring even though the content in very stimulating. It's the monotone voice that makes them think the presentation is dull. So as speakers we must be concerned with exhibiting the appropriate tone of voice for our content and have the appropriate tone for the message we want to communicate. See if your teacher has spent any time learning how to effectively communicate and teach instead of just showing off what they are regurgitating.

Many times a yoga teacher stays safe and just repeats what they have learned in school or seen or heard others do and say. Your teacher should start there, but find ways to create their own unique teaching method and choose what exactly they want to share. I find that the old advertising and political slogan, 'keep it simple stupid,' perpetrates stupidity. You are not stupid and do not want to feel that way in a public yoga class. I have sat in on classes where the teacher demeans and talks down to their students as if they are some all-knowing oracle. I have also endured hours of too much talking trying to explain everything the teacher knows in an hour. For me, finding a balance of what to share, how to educate a student effectively, seeing where they are at in their understanding, making sure you are heard and sharing something unique or new creates an enriched learning environment.

Stand Out

Even when I was starting out and teaching just classes in the gym and fitness world I tried to do something that was unique to the gym classes. I started class with a breathing exercise, which I have heard many teachers do not do at the gym, but regardless of where it is taught, breathing is the foundation of Yoga and we are not really doing Yoga if we are not breathing properly. So I do it anyway. I liked to explain that a Mudra is a sacred hand gesture with a purpose. When you reach for something over head on a shelf you reach with strength and intention. I would explain the energy involved in moving our arm, and ask why we do a weak armed overhead reach in a yoga posture? It is a challenge as an instructor to know when to stop speaking and just let some in the class do the postures incorrectly. That explains why when I take some peoples classes the instructor just says three or four generic instructions and then are quiet and half the class is doing the posture incorrectly and potentially hurting themselves. The instructor has not determined if their message was heard and received by their students and if not, how could they improve.

After making the decision to step away from 'fitness Yoga' and seek out a better understanding of the transformation I could feel my body and mind going through, I did what I always do, I researched. I am a 'feet in first' kind of person. Having never been a runner, I decided to run two full marathons. I get obsessive when I am fully committed. yoga was the same. Once I committed to finding the authentic teacher, I jumped in. I had parameters; they had to be originally from India, they had to be alive, they had to have achieved an amount of recognition and they had to be accessible for a reasonable amount of money. As I typed in 'Yoga Guru's' in Google a huge amount of information came up. Being me, I started at the top and skimmed down, looking for a feeling. Deepak Chopra had always intrigued me. He had a facility close; he went on the list. Self-Realization Fellowship is close, but they are not really teaching Yoga anymore, Yogi Amrit Desai, never heard of him but whoa! As his picture came up, I felt a surge in my heart, my mouth formed a grin, I got a tickle in my chest...but wait, he was located all the way in Florida. Back to Deepak, he is closer, but no feeling.

I looked up when a class was being held at the center and decided to attend to see what I could find out. The chase was on; I was on the trail of a Guru. What I found was a seasoned experienced teacher who could handle almost any question from a variety of students' backgrounds and experiences with efficiency and ease.

Observe your teacher, are they in 'thinking and doing' mode, looking around the room at others, worrying if they have right and left sorted out, analyzing what is going on and getting lost in the over thinking mind? Is that the appropriate mode for the stage of the posture that you are in? If not, can your teacher and leader, guide you into a more passive and feeling place taking the emphasis off the technical and into the inner domain? As the leader, are they working from the students and the feedback they are getting? What exactly are you needing at this point in the posture for it to be a transformative experience? A master teacher will take the leadership role and meet them where they are at. The teacher will coach students to a better understanding of how to execute the posture and have a transformation in it. The expression on the students face when it shifts from confusion and frustration, to an understanding is the quickening of their inner connection to self. You can sense that they have just experienced an 'Aha' moment about their own body. Many of us inhabit the body for centuries before beginning self-exploration. Self-exploration, be it physical, mental, emotional, spiritual or intellectual is the key to having a Yogic transformative experience.

Bad Ass Yoga

One of the questions I ask when interviewing potential teachers is, "Why do you want to be a teacher?" Then I listen. I am listening for answers that talk about the student, not the teacher. If all I hear as an answer is I, I, I, they have missed the point. Teaching is leading, being a student is surrendering to the path the teacher is taking you on. Both take a great amount of dedication and trust. Are you someone the students can trust and will listen to? Where are you leading your students? Is it a rambling road with lots of stops along the way Is it a challenging steep climb with rock to traverse, or is it a straight and direct path to the results? Are you there for them should they fall? Do you know what your student's fears and limitations are? No one likes a dictator (unless you're a Bikram student). We all want to follow someone whom we trust will lead us to a place we want to go safely and in due time. Be the leader for your students' transformation.

A teacher should not be selling, or performing and the class should not be about them. The teacher should be based in a long lineage of teachers, not corporate yoga training. A teacher who makes up an intention about their own needs is not considering the student. I do not set an intention for the student but encourage them to discover their own by asking themselves Why? Why are they there. A lineage of teachers who are grounded and loving will create an entirely different experience for their students compared to a celebrity teacher who is there to self-serve. Is the teacher serving up a big fat serving of their ego or looking to help the student? Is the teacher trying to be bad ass, only wanting to be in a bad ass class, teaching bad ass students in their bad ass yoga clothes? Bad-Ass-Yoga.

A master teacher should be inviting students into sanctuary, a sanctuary the teacher has built to share with them. A yoga class can be a chance to escape from daily lives. A retreat for the student from the action and activity of the day. For this hour you should get to leave life's challenges at the door, or privately bring them in to work through. The class, in my world, should be a place you can sigh as you enter and relax your shoulders and heart. A vacation from whatever is on their plate for the day/ week/ life ahead. In order to let ourselves as students completely relax and have a transformative experience, we have to trust the teacher. We need to know that we are safe, in a loving environment with other likeminded people. If we feel fear, pressure, or unsafe by the teacher's manners, we cannot trust and cannot retreat. A master teacher should create a sanctuary of trust and invite their students in.

Authenticity

The authentic teacher I found inspiration and learning in is Yogi Amrit Desai. Four years after I met my teacher, he came for a public talk at my studio! So many people that I have shared his teachings with were able to hear his words. I was in bliss and ecstasy. When Yogi Amrit Desai came to the studio for 'The Urge to Merge' workshop, I noticed his photo which I always have out, and then looked over to see him sitting next to me. I was tickled with bliss. My teacher, who has illuminated my life and whose words and teachings take me to the light of the understanding, had taught me as his student. I shared in my own humble manner what I learned from him with the students. This is the lineage of teaching. Full circle. I watched when he was at my studio as others laughed out loud at his unique mix of insight and humor (I am so glad that my teacher has a sense of humor). I was thrilled to see others taking notes, hearing the truth in the message. I delighted when others eyes glimpsed over at me and twinkled. I floated on a cloud I thought was a cushion under me as I looked up at my teacher. No saint, but a man; a man who has suffered life's ups and downs and stayed in the light of teaching others. This is what teaching was about. I was so proud he was in the Yoga studio and that by sharing his teachings it allowed me to educate and illuminate others. The right teacher will speak the truth to you. You will know it when you hear it. I empower you to not take less or endure a teacher that is not striving for their best. Even my teacher at one point had to seek out and find his teacher.

The Making of a teacher. A story of my teachers' teacher.

My teacher, Amrit Desai, found his teacher, or his teacher found him, when he was a very young man. His teachers name was Swami Kripalavanandaji or Bapuji as he was affectionately called. Babuji was completely and entirely dedicated to his quest of knowledge, education and teaching others. During a very important stage in his knowledge through experience, Bapuji changed his diet completely during his first year of Yogic meditation. Each day he ate only a couple of spoonful's of ground peanuts with sugar and a few spoonful's of vegetables, usually potatoes. Twice: a day he drank hot milk diluted with water. He lost a lot of weight. Once, Bapuji wandered away from Rijpipla. In a transcendental state of spiritual bliss, wearing no clothes, he visited several villages, on foot. People from Mota Fofatia (a local" village) heard about this. They were devotees of Bapuji. Realizing that this naked saint was Bapuji, they ran to him to take him to their village. Because he wouldn't sleep at night and might wander off, devotees stayed up to keep a constant watch. Yet one night he dodged them and stole off to another village, Kanjetha. The devotees of Kanjetha found him and took him to stay near a temple on the banks of the river Narmada. After hours of sitting in bliss, he suddenly got up and plunged into the strong currents of the Narmada. The river flowed fast and strong during the month of Shraavan (the monsoon season). Soon- he was in midstream. The river looked as if it would sweep him away. The night was pitch dark. The Narmada was furious and powerful during the rainy season. Anxious devotees swung their lanterns from side to side, searching tearfully. One of them said, "We are not helping Bapuji by crying. Let us move ahead along the bank. In a couple of hours, it will be dawn. Perhaps there will be some ray of hope for us then." Everyone agreed that it was a good idea. They started running along the bank, their lanterns moving like fireflies.

Bapuji continued to swim for some 'time but eventually exhaustion set in." For several days he had eaten and slept little. His long hike had weakened him immensely. He was drained of all physical energy. It was a miracle that he was swimming at all. As his hands and feet became numb with fatigue, he cried out in prayer to his teacher: "Gurudev, I am drowning ... help me ... save me ... " Suddenly Dadaji's voice broke through the torrent of raging sound. "Give up Swimming, Stop Swimming" Bapuji's body was completely exhausted. Often he was swept down into the surging waters. His mind was snapping. He had lost all sense of time and space. Dadaji's words came to him fuzzily, as if they were echoes of his imagination. He kept swimming. then he heard the voice again: "Swami! Stop swimming; surrender:' Now there was no doubt about it. He knew that it was his beloved Gurdev speaking. It was his familiar voice. It was no fiction. A great and triumphant feeling of courage and bliss swept through him and his arms and legs stopped moving. Then there was a miracle. His body became light and floated on the surface of the water while he relaxed completely. His fears of drowning left him. Unknowingly, he chanted this mantra:

OM NAMAH SHIVA Y GURAVE SATCHITANAND MURTA YE; NAMASTA SMA " NA MAS TA SMA I, NAMASTASMA I, NAMO NAMAH.

(0 Lord Shiva, I bow to Thee in the blissful form of the Guru; To Thee I bow, to Thee I bow, to Thee I bow respectfully.)

His body floated gently in the water like a flower, at times near one bank and at times near the other, often in midstream. A couple of hours later he reached Sinor Village, on the shore. It was morning and the sun shone brightly. The search party of devotees found him and joyfully shouted, "Long live Gurudev!" Their joyful shouting echoed all along the shore. Bapuji swam toward them and came out of the water, smiling. All of them collapsed in tears of joy. Through Dadaji's infinite grace and power, Bapuji left the black and swirling river safely. - Yogi Amrit Desai.

A teacher is doing Karma Yoga, the Yoga of service. How is the teacher showing up to serve the student? They should be a leader. The teacher should know where they are taking them and lead them with confidence. A great teacher should sit with their students, breathe with them, be their friend. A yoga teacher needs to center themselves and their students often. Think through the posture sequence with a purpose and let the student know what lies ahead. Love their students, which is why the teacher is there! The teacher is their students lifeguard, keeping them safe. A master teacher remembers the vast and different ways others learn. Everyone learns differently. Some are more auditory, visual, or kinesthetic. A true teacher allows the student to shine, but ask all egos and inner critics to wait outside during practice.

CHAPTER SIX
Will I become a hippy?

"My mother used to say "Take a deep Breath".
I was too busy to give any real thought to what she was
trying to teach me.
Years have passed and Yoga is teaching me what she meant
all along. Pause, reflect, breathe.
Balance and flexibility; It carries itself into everyday in every
season.
There is more to life than increasing its speed."
Mahatma Ghandi

'Inhale rainbows, exhale unicorns'. I often joke about the
yoga voice many teachers adopt and the false persona of a perfected
master. It is not realistic to me to think that yoga will suddenly bring
enlightenment or solve all of our problems. There are many
moments of joy and bliss, a sense of union and oneness that happen
in yoga. A community if formed and people begin to see how
connected we all are. A yoga class is a journey that we all go one
together leaving us with a feeling of being a part of a tribe or group
of people who have just gone through an experience together. Once
we redirect our attention on a new and positive habit consistently,
the old ways and habits will slowly begin to fade away. In the
Pramahansa Yogananda movie Awake the teacher is telling a
follower that his teachings will not make a student stop smoking or
drinking but those habits will leave them the more they follow his
teachings. One of the reasons I started to deepen my yogic studies
was to find the answer to the questions my students kept asking.

Most often when someone was new I would introduce myself and let them know they could ask me any questions along their path. If they practiced consistently, they would start to notice changes. Yoga teaches our body, on a subtle level to stretch, elongate, lighten and stand tall. The nervous system begins to reset and release spontaneously pent up tension and stress. Then they would ask if I knew why they felt so much better and how come things were healing for them. I knew I needed to deepen my understanding to answer their questions.

I have witnessed many transformations during the years of teaching thousands of students. Often, students will release with a loud cry or moan. I remember in a hot yoga studio in the traditional method in a famous Southern California beach town, I let out a moan. The teacher laughed over the loud speaker at the sound my spontaneous release made. Then commented to all to hear that obviously it was camel pose but that we did not need to make any camel sounds in the pose. My classes are the opposite of that approach. I actually encourage students to release in class. To move on their own without direction in postures or in repose. I feel satisfied when a student is in a posture and follows their bodies to the sound of their own drummer. Just like I did in Camel Pose, many people had their hearts opened in class. I encourage socializing before and after class and people created life long bonds and friendships.

Opening your heart can mean many things. We can try to do it alone, but often it requires being receptive to accepting love and intimacy from another. We can find the trust to allow our heart to open. Once the trust in ourselves has been encouraged, we can eventually allow our heart to remain open even in stressful situations that life presents, disagreements with others, and life's challenges.

As we work on physical, mental and emotional tools that help us to stay open, we may even begin to understand empathy.

Devotion

In Sanskrit, the term Bhakti translates into a devotional relationship on a personal level with the student's self, their teacher and for some their relationship with creation. The fastest way to a deeper relationship with life and the world is devotional love. There are many different paths, of course, and no hierarchy is formed for different paths. It is just believed by practicing the yoga of devotion, a student's path to union is expedited. This is not to be taken lightly as a serious devotion of love is the most binding relationship one can be blessed to have. Usually, the relationship is between a teacher and a student. Having a living master to learn from is ideal as you can have questions answered and mysteries solved for you as the student. One line of teachers is traced back from teacher to master for generations. So as the wisdom is passed from teacher to teacher it is passed from generation to generation. When you feel a part of a movement, it is usually centered in your heart.

I remember saying once to my teacher, that I had never thought I could feel as close to another guy like I did for my father. The father and son bond is unique and sacred. I realized after a while of studying the Amrit method that I could see a difference between the teacher and the man. When I related to him as a down to earth human who was blessed with being a teacher, but nevertheless, a man living his life, I realized that I was a bhakti yogi. I was blessed in this life to feel like my teacher was also a father figure and I could devote my practice to the teachings of his lineage. It gave my practice a sense of being grounded in a tradition. The acceptance and friendships formed are lifelong. My heart was opened at one training and I thought, this is it, the reason so many have been doing yoga. Once a heart is opened it can never be closed again.

One day of training at the ashram, I told my teacher that I finally understood what empathy meant after hearing all the sharing after class. Everyone laughed at my comment, thinking I was joking, so I laughed along. I was serious though. I was just beginning to understand what having my heart opened meant. I could not imagine not having the experience I was having. I could actually and physically feel my heart opening to others after hearing them share their stories. I went from thinking that others all had perfect lives and only mine had so much struggle, to seeing that I had so much to be thankful for. My struggles have never been as hard as some others.

Having my heart opened through yoga, meditation and living my teacher's teachings I felt called to serve others. I opened my own yoga studio to give to others. My feeling of connection to others and life in general deepened. I started also wanting to learn more myself and take care of my health. Once my heart opened, much to my surprise, I felt like all I wanted to do was help others in any way I could. It was during a deep meditation led by my teacher that I got the idea for opening a studio. Four years of being voted the best studio in town by the citizens confirmed the value that giving has. I was aware of how I affect others or am affected by others state of being. We are all connected, biologically if you are science minded or on deeper energy levels if your belief system allows. It can make us become aware of how our actions, thoughts, words and deeds influence our outside world and our internal landscape.

Where is Your Heart Located?

The physical body is the location of the muscle called the heart. Located inside bone, ribs and a shield called the sternum, it is cradled by connective tissue, muscles, and virtually ignored and unacknowledged by its owner. Ask most people to put their hands over their heart and they will place them in the middle of their chest rather than the actual physical location.

As you place the hands over the heart you can feel it shielded by armor; physical, mental and emotional armor. Often more than not, the armor is layered by years and years of physical tension, emotional scars, hurts and angers. When we have suppressed hurt and anger it is physically impossible, on our own, to open our heart. In yoga, we do physical postures or stretches to open the heart and it hurts, our shoulders are rounded forward and our backs hurt. Most humans mentally try to deal with life's ups and downs, using the mind as the foraging tool. To release tension, often times we need the help of another, but first we have to trust them, and that takes a lot of letting go. Sometimes just the right person in the form of a teacher comes along and their open heart pulls at ours until we just give in.

Physically we can learn breathing exercises, we can do stretches, we can try Yoga and see if that helps. Mentally we can try to stay busy all the time, racing from one thing to the other, staying constantly busy and amplifying the chatter to drown out the hurting in the heart. But emotionally, we need that trust and another person to show us the way, to make us feel safe enough to go inside and begin to melt the armor. That can get tricky if we are just relying on a lover to be our counselor. Often times after the newness of a relationship wears off and people reveal who they really are beyond the falling in love farce, the hurts are revealed. It takes a special kind of love and partner to help fix the other. Often times, the work to heal or deal with what is in the heart, in any relationship, takes its toll. Many relationships cannot weather the healing that most of us need. The relationship dissolves and the partners think to themselves that they will watch out and try to not get someone with 'that' problem in the next partner. But the next partner has some other thing that takes special care to fix.

A friend is so invested, too, that we risk pushing them away. The friend knows us too well and often will not let their friend complain much. A true friend though will guide someone needing healing to the right teacher. A mentor, coach or teacher (called Guru in Yoga) is often the only way we can confront what we don't even know we are burying. Most of us are here needing some sort of self-development work. I know for me meeting my teacher, Amrit Desai, and his staff, which includes his beautiful daughter Kamini Desai, has forever changed my life. His life's teachings and work and the resource of his teacher from India on the reactive mind is a panacea for most of what is ailing society and us its citizens. Through his teachings I am, how to manage the crazy mind. I practice how to love my self just as I am including without judgement. My 'faults' led me to this place of helping others like I never imagined would be possible.

Finding the right teaching has helped Jenny Plantz discover her 'Why' of yoga: *"Yoga, for me, has been a transformational journey. Over the years, I have had a variety of teachers; from veterans to rookies, young, old, conservative and radical, I feel blessed to have experienced such diversity. When I look at how dramatically my life has changed since I started practicing yoga, I see how influential my yoga teachers have been. Often the most profound experiences take time to unfold and process before I realize how significant they are. A seemingly simple comment a teacher made in class may pop back into my mind and guide me when I am dealing with some form of struggle in my daily life; this the mark of a great teacher. They bestow these wonderful gifts when you are on the mat and then, at the most challenging times, you discover that you have the tools you need to press through the trials of life gracefully. So, in gratitude for the wonderful gifts my teachers have selflessly given me, I aim toward the same goal; to uplift, inspire, strengthen, open up, and connect with those who are close to me. I am becoming a yoga teacher to give back to others all that I have been given."*

Once you have found a way to open your heart, you will begin to want to take care of it. Just to be clear, you can approach this from the biological viewpoint. Opening the physical structure, the ribs, connective tissue and stretching the abdominal muscles to allow your body to expand and breathe deeper has wonderful health benefits. Physically you will naturally want to breathe deep more often after doing yoga breath work. This will get a student in touch with their cardio vascular system and how it functions to retrieve oxygen to the body for health. The student then will want to keep their lungs healthy and perhaps learn how to eat healthier for their heart health and longevity.

Some students will want to use a more emotional approach to this feeling of having their heart lightened through the less physical elements of yoga. These students may place hands on heart and feel layers upon layers of armor. They may want to try taking a deep breath into their hands, filling them with love, turning them outward and sending the love out to the universe. They may be looking for a deeper connection to that which they believe they were before this body and that which might survive after the body. Either way most of us could listen to our heart and let it guide us to the right teacher/ teachers that will help (sometimes force) us to unlock the armor and breath freely again.

For many, "opening your heart" implies receptivity to love and intimacy in a romantic relationship—bring on the candy and flowers. However, everyone, including single yoga practitioners, can experience heart opening in other kinds of relationships: with caring friends and family members, pets, teachers and mentors, and with our own students. With deep introspection and honesty, you can also practice heart opening in more challenging situations, such as your relationships with difficult people or those with whom you disagree philosophically or politically. As you visualize and practice opening your heart in your various relationships, you're learning ahimsa, or compassion, which is number one on the list of Yamas and Niyamas.

Find the Heart Space

The physical location of the heart is within the skeletal and muscular system of the body, locked in a protective chamber of the strongest material the body can produce. A cage of ribs surrounds the area of the heart. A core of tissue and muscle hide the pump of the body. Bone is connected with super strong tendons that link the sepulcher of the heart together. Some feel their emotions and anxiety in this physical place. Others are vaguely aware that the heart if keeping the life flowing through their veins. A unique and highly functional muscle spans below the heart, running horizontal, that creates the final layer of protection around our most vital organ.

When the body is stretched, moved and used, the encasing of the heart is soft and pliable. When the body breathes in the tissue surrounding the heart opens and expands. It is equivalent to wearing your favorite sweater. As your breath the sweater is just the right size to expand a little and still remain comfortable. However, once washed in hot water and dried on high heat, the sweater becomes too snug. It simply will not stretch like it did before its shrinking. It is no longer comfortable when you try to breathe. It simply has become stiff and will not move. Over time, the unmoved, aging or ill body reacts the same way. It stiffens and wont expand, thus cutting off slowly the source of all life, the oxygen that keeps the heart beating. Yoga keeps the body moving and free, allowing more access to the heart, health and freedom of movement. I recently had a flair up from my old neck injury and the pain was immeasurable. One morning I awoke to find my head would not go straight over my neck. The muscle spasm was so intense that my body had frozen in place. The pain lasted for six weeks around my thoracic spine. The area that needs to expand was locked tight. I could feel over the weeks that my breathing was constricted and I could not do my daily deep breathing exercises. My daily stress and tension accumulated and I found it very hard to deal with stress without being able to breath. Back pain and tension can cause anyone to begin to lose health. There is a whole branch of yoga which focuses on breathing techniques. These techniques, many of which are taught best in various forms from a living teacher keep the body moveable and breathable.

Heart Opening Yoga Sequence by Shanti Troy

*Ask your medical professional before trying any new physical activity. Use your best judgement. Take the time to look up each of these postures on line, watch my You Tube video that matches this series or email me for details and practice each one individually with safety and your limitations in mind before linking together into a sequence. Start by closing your eyes, slowing your breath and checking in. How are you feeling physically, mentally, emotionally and otherwise? Just note the state you are in without doing anything to change or fix it. Make a mental note.

- **Seated Back Bend**
- **Cat/ Cow/Down Dog**
- **War. I, Wide Arm Stance**
- **Wide Arm Chair**
- **War II/ Side Angle Bound/ Rev. Warrior**
- **Eagle/Open arm Chair/ Eagle/ Open Arm Mountain**
- **Dancers Posture**
- **Chest Expansion**
- **Cobra/ Bound Cobra**
- **Seated Forward Fold**
- **Bridge/ Wheel**
- **Shoulder Stand**
- **Corpse Posture**

After the sequence, pause with the eyes close and notice if there is any difference in your thoughts, words, actions or deed towards yourself mentally, emotionally, physically or otherwise.

Opening your heart can mean many things. We can try to do it alone, but often it requires being receptive to accepting love and intimacy from another. Intimate, or with friends, family members, teachers, and with even strangers, we can find the trust to allow our heart to open. Once the trust in ourselves has been encouraged, we can eventually allow our heart to remain open even in stressful situations that life presents. As we work on physical, mental and emotional tools that help us to stay open we may even begin to understand empathy. Feeling our own life's experience deeper and having empathy for others journey may create the sense of having an 'open heart.' This feeling of connectedness to your own fragility and others plights may make you act more compassionate. Often I find students happier after class. If encouraged, after yoga class conversations are often the best. Students smile, laugh and relate with each other after class. I love the feeling of community that can be generated in the yoga environment. This feeling of love and closeness could be attributed to the 'hippy' population. Either way, you may begin to feel healthier, happier and concerned more for the wellbeing of others when yoga opens your heart. If you feel resistant to connecting on a deeper to others, ask yourself why. Where is the resistance coming from? In yoga, we like to observe our triggers or reactions but we do not need to try and fix them, or judge ourselves. We simply witness what is causing a road block and observe how we are with it. As an introvert, it is easy for me to keep a wall up and stay disconnected. Yoga recognizes the place in us where we each meet. It shines a light on our similarities. If I can recognize attributes and qualities in others that I also possess, the gap of differences will be bridged and I will only begin to see how we are all similar. Traveling to India, and the tiny mud village my teacher grew up in was just a small stop on our trip. However, the happiness in the children, playing in the dirt with sticks and each other profoundly changed my life. I handed out candied ginger and they acted as though I was giving out gold pieces. They did not fight with each other, but patiently waited for me to place a candy in their hand. The smiling faces and out stretched arms and pure joy within them radiating out opened my heart to how similar we all are. I will remember that second in my life of pure bliss and joy in the simplest act of handing out candy for all existence. I can still see their huge grins, hands opened, hearts connected permanently etched into the fiber of my being. That second of pure heart opening, simplicity and connectedness of these little Indian children and a boy from Kansas over giving and receiving was yoga, union, heart opening. There is no greater joy than no words, just a simple smile and gratitude. Only yoga, union, could have given me this moment and I could never have experienced it without an open heart.

CHAPTER SEVEN
Why should I meditate?

"There is more to life than increasing its speed."
Mahatma Gandhi

Meditation, known in the yoga world as Yoga Nidra, is nothing mystical or magical and can be approached by anyone from any cultural background. It can be supported and broken down by science in understanding that the brain operates on many different brain waves. Different brain waves are for different purposes. One can easily learn to guide their own mind or be led by a teacher into a more relaxed state of mind. Mountains of time have been dedicated over centuries to the pursuit of meditation. The first step I approach the subject with is to speak of the medical and neurological effects of meditation. The parasympathetic and the sympathetic nervous systems service two different functions of the body and brain.

A part of the brain that can be trained to respond and repeat even while awake may be accessed by the parasympathetic nervous system in meditation. By mastering the body, the brain can be formed to function the way the meditator wants it to. Meditation teaches you to not react to old programming that no longer serves your needs. Learning to not react, the nervous system is able to relax and conserve nervous system energy. The meditator can learn to control the body's energy and direct it to areas on command. Mediation has such a lengthy history and many well documented personal accounts of the positive benefits; it could be called irrefutable. Many have written how that for them meditation can create a sense of calm mind or mindfulness, the stress on the body reduces naturally and a pleasant approach to life can begin with meditation practice. As always I find if I share a personal experience and my own techniques it resonates more than simply disseminating information.

What Can Meditation Do for Me?

Yoga Nidra (sleep yoga or meditation) can enhance the healing process and boost the immune system. It is effective in helping with stress, addictions, sleep disorders, nervous conditions and in releasing long-standing behavioral patterns. How we cope with and respond to stress changes. Recently I was tested by two unrelated individuals who showed me their true nature of chaos and anger. In both of these unfortunate situations, I called upon my breathing skills and meditative focus. By recognizing myself in a threatening situation I was able to call on my years of meditation and breathing training and not meet these individuals at their anger level. It can actually be quite amazing and funny to watch as others have a moment of breaking their façade and showing who they really are inside from a meditative perspective. We are emotional creatures and it takes much work and training to rise above survival emotions. I have found through meditation and teaching it to others, many approaches to life have shifted and changed.

Teachers always like to remind us that learning about a subject in a book is not the same as the lesson learned from the experience of living and surviving the subject. I have experiences all the time that remind me of how meditation has helped me personally. I had a situation unfold once that greatly called upon my training. It all began when I found out that my landlord was being foreclosed on, and I would have to move. This was during the housing market collapse and was my second landlord to give up their condo. I guess at the height of the market anyone could 'own' a condo. Up to this point I had only once rented from a corporation. I had always rented from private home owners. Moving out in ten days is not easy and I could not have done it without the help of some friends and clients. Thank God for the help. This particular condo though, I had come quit attached to. I lived next to a friend, it was in my favorite location for walking and I had begun the process of trying to buy my first home. Often I found myself thinking, "I teach stress reduction, I can do this." Then I got sick. It was what I thought was the worst flu I ever got. Traditionally I heal myself, but this was only getting worse, so upon visiting the doctor I found out I was one week away from having pneumonia. Medication, teaching yoga, personal training, sleeping on couches, I realize is small in the arena of homelessness, but it was the first time I felt without a home or a plan.

Reflecting, the only things that kept me together, positive and calm were the techniques I have learned since studying stress management. I often speak about these techniques to others in my attempts to be inspirational, I read about them, listen to my teacher's teachings, but rarely do I get to practice them as fully as I did in those few months of being forced out of a home I wanted to stay in for a long time and possibly own. Many times I share my stress dealing tips with others, but never have to practice them myself. Meditation has taught me to deal with situations head on. In my family, when we have conflict, we deal with it right then and there, even if it involves heated words, and passionate feelings. Then we resolve it and move on. We try to let it go and not let it linger on and on. I have to realize; some people do not deal with conflict this way. Some run away from it and never resolve it. We have three choices, fight, flight, or deal. When we can deal with the situation at hand, talk it out, find a solution, it can be released and resolved. I always remember the saying, it is not what happens to us, it is how we deal with it. Dealing with it is the only way to not carry it around, suppress it and have it manifest later. So with each thing that came up for me, I tried to confront it, resolve it and move on, not put it off until later, run away or ignore it and hope it would go away on its own.

Shake it off. Easy said, how to do? Familiarize yourself with your anatomical and biological body. Research the nervous system and its different systems. Once aware of our body and how it functions, you can begin to use the mind to manage it at will. I call it mind management, though others have told me that sounds a little culty, it works for me. One of the greatest mediation techniques that have stuck with me is so simple yet effective. Perceive your body as a factory. You are managing a city. The body has its energy requirements to function, it has a fuel processing center, waste management, a central command center with a super computer overseeing and running the entire facility. The name of the factory is your name, or whatever you want to call yourself. The product this factory makes are the thoughts, words, actions and deeds that you produce. I know this seems a little rudimentary. The way it has helped me the most though as a meditative tool, is to know or believe that 'I' am in control of that factory and make the decisions that need to be made. I then look at the nervous system as a mechanical function that I oversee. It moves the primal from functioning on its own to being a service that you can manage. If you notice that the body or mind is responding to stress in a biological way you can stop it. Noticing that the heart rate is increasing and the pupils are dilating from stress, the breath is becoming short and staccato can alert you that your body is about to enter flight and fight. In a conflict, usually the primal flight or fight reaction does not lead to a peaceful and productive solution. If you are viewing your body as a factory, you can command the nervous system to relax, and override the cardio vascular system to remain calm and peaceful even in the face of someone yelling at you.

Look at nervous or scared animals. Their nervous systems take over and shake the stress out of their body. As humans we have to convince the mind to relinquish control of the body and allow us to, 'shake it off.'   There is a ton of research to support this simple idea. We can release physical stress caused by situations in life through physical activity. Unresolved stress, stuffed down and repressed can manifest as illness, emotional blockages that resurface later, and result in repeating the same patterns of destructive behavior and required counseling. In Yoga we call it Samskara. For me it is my Yoga physical practice that releases stress in my body, joints, muscles, and mind. For others it is running, boxing, dancing, swimming, or weight lifting. Whatever activity you can find, shake it off. Get it out of your mind for an hour, build up heat that burns out stress, get a massage, get it out of the physical body. The best I felt during challenging times was after teaching/ doing a very vigorous yoga class. In balance postures, our minds simply cannot think of anything else but being in the present moment, or we fall over.

Another technique I like to utilize even while in the midst of a stressful situation is to imagine what the situation would look like if written it down. This is one I do not practice enough, but over the stressful times, it has been a lifesaver. Picturing how this situation would look later in writing minimizes the immediateness of whatever stress it is. I actually keep a note pad by the bed with a pen, and make it the only thing on the night stand. Every night just before falling asleep write down the scenario that caused you stress that day, set it aside, do not annualize it, and then close your eyes and let it go. This way, you get out of your head, worrying about what you have to do the next day, or about what you did not get done. It simply cannot sit there as you are trying to sleep and roll around in your mind. It is out of you and on a physical piece of paper. The next morning reviews your writing, more likely than not, that situation will seem significantly less important and a solution may even appear to make it go away.

Take a breath. Think about the last time you felt really relaxed. Maybe at the end of yoga or meditation. Bringing to mind the way this felt, even in the midst of a major stressor is so effective. It really is the one technique to learn. You need to create the muscle memory of actually having experienced deep relaxation to draw upon the feeling. It cannot be faked. You must create moments of conscious deep awareness in your life. Taking a yoga class can create this feeling even in the most basic gym yoga class. You should feel the joy in a natural bliss state and store that memory to conjure up later. Finding the right amount of time to rest the body, rest the mind, rest the heart. Being a type A, I always want to go the extra mile and believe sleep is for when I am in the grave, but under times of stress, the body and mind need to sleep, plain and simple, sleep heals all. The first thing the doctor said to me was go home and sleep. Boy was he right. I hope these fairly simple techniques help you someday, that your life is free of stress and that you can sleep.

One of the best ways to remember how joy feels is a simple technique that I often start class with. Relaxing the body and mind and feeling safe allows one to lower their guard. Once the mind and body feel safe and relaxed one can become aware of the mood or state of mind. Being aware of the current state of emotions created by the mind we can contemplate the idea that we can control the up and downs of the mind and moods that so often steal our energy and attention. Closing the eyes removes the stimulation of the senses. Once a person feels centered, calm, safe and in control they can elicit change by choice. Using memory and the realistic trigger response it creates, we can remind ourselves of a person, place or thing that brings us pure joy. Feel that place, person or thing in detail. The smell, mood, feeling, temperature, recreating it as realistically in your mind's eye as you possible can. Truly experience it. Notice how you feel once you open your eyes again. You control the mind and emotions at will, they do not control you. You can create this at will. You are your own best teacher.

What can a meditation teacher do for me?

Once a person has witnessed something greater than the mind, greater than the body, an awareness that there is something more to us than just the physical, they can do one of two things. They can dive in to the awareness and work on living in the moment and developing the awareness that we are much more then we think or fight against it. When I saw the saint Amma for the first time, I felt my whole awareness shift suddenly and unexpectedly. I stood out on the edge of the universe, surrounded in a shroud of stars, I felt Amma's presence surrounding me in safety as I sat on the precipice of our solar system and the presence of my friend who got the hug with me. I could see stretched out before me, the entire solar system of this galaxy. The lights were so immense and the vastness so overwhelming that I felt I could not breathe. But Amma's loving presence kept me safe. I could see the entire solar system in front of me yet I felt safe. A knowingness descended upon me. I felt as if data was being downloaded to me that we are of the universe and will return to the universe. I understood that we are all made of the universal material and will one-day return to that universal matter again. I took mantra meditation and used her prescribed mantra for a year in my meditations.

The knowledge I gained from that one brief sight Amma's hug revealed to me has continued to digest to this date. We are all one, of the same material, to return to that material again one day. Made of the same matter as all living beings, plant animal, matter and metal. I have had the realization that we are one with all things, beings and matter in this universe. At once, most feel they then need to become falsely spiritual with this advice. It is however important to realize through your own deductions, that this world is all the same matter, exchanging, manifesting, dissolving and returning again and again. Most of you, the body and brain, are made of matter that has existed for centuries, just being reassembled. What we see as our lives, our vital likes and dislikes, what we hold to be of such importance on this planet, is really a speck of dust on the timeline of the universe. All this matter has circulated and been reformed for eons. It is just a temporary blip on the timeline of all that matters. But for this time, we occupy this matter now. We choose, or it was chosen for us, to manifest into this matter we are in that we call 'us.' Whether Amma did anything to me or I placed myself in the right position for my own learning is debatable. Placing myself in the teacher's arena though caused me to have these perspectives that have changed my view of reality as it shows up in my life. I have had many life perspective shifts happen in my searching and seeking for master teachers. The teacher can create the environment for the student to shift into a meditative state easier.

The Amrit yoga teacher training program is deeper and more profound than I ever expected. I learned more in the first four days than I have learned in all my yoga trainings. There is something to say for learning from the direct source. On the day we received an energy transference from Amrit that was more intense and all-encompassing than I can even begin to describe. I felt pain, ecstasy, love and fear all simultaneously. There are not words big or illustrious enough to describe what happened. I just know I will never be the same, never see the world the same and none of my classes will ever be the same. I only hope I can bring a glimmer of the light I saw that day to everyone in my life and not be taken out of the light.

Brain vs Mind

Death meditation is a Yoga technique. Bhagavan Das described in his autobiography being taught the fragility of life by meditating at the funeral pyres in India where bodies are cremated. The mediator is covered by ash from the fires of the bodies and drink from a skull cap. The actual top of a scull is their cup and dinner plate. As primitive and blunt as this appears it is a stark way of seeing the fragility of life and the distinction of mind from brain and body. You can also achieve this when someone close to you dies and at least for my obsessive mind, the survivor contemplates the horrible things your loved one went through in dying and what their body must be doing as the years go by. The practice of burial in a coffin with embalming is preposterous and polluting. The body is filed with chemicals to prevent decay and stuck in a very expensive box that won't decompose. So the body never gets to return to earth or nature. It's a superstitious practice. I'd rather return to ash. And if you contemplate for a spell what happens to the body in cremation you can't be attached either. However instead of meditation on death I feel the same result can be achieved by contemplating on the miraculous functioning of the body we inhabit. The visceral effect of being inside a machine such as the physical and being aware of its biology reminds me that I am not this body and that it's biology is finite in its functioning. It then becomes an invaluable and irreplaceable commodity that one has to care for and maintain the best one can while in possession of it. Just contemplating the chemistry of the sperm and its miraculous journey to fertilize the egg that become the body reveals the fragility of our bodies and shows us how it takes biological matter that existed before we became conscious to create that which we call 'Our Body.' How did it become ours? Did we purchase it? No. It was a gift to us to care for and maintain while in possession of it. Or it is in possession of us. It needs an operating system to run it efficiently. The brain is the hard drive and the operating system is our consciousness.

The mind is our knowledge our self-identity what we have learned in our life, our family traits and heritage. Our brain is an organ, tissue and matter controlling and regulating the functions of the body. It keeps the body in balance through chemistry. We need it to be healthy so we can enjoy a well-functioning machine. It has to work optimally with the body and other organs. But it's not our ego mind which contains our thoughts, learned behavior and intellect. So I've been working on staying out of my mind and focusing on the brains function and relationship with the rest of the body. These ideas are why eating disorders are a mental illness. The brain doesn't want the body abused for if there is no body there is no brain. Learning the physical damage caused by starvation, dehydration or over eating is eye opening and sometimes irreversible. If we eat for healthy function of the brain and body, we then lose unhealthy habits and learned behavior eating that may cause the body harm. Most all religions and higher practices suggest forms of abstaining from that which in excess can cause the body harm. Intoxicant distractions that potentially numb the mind but destroy the body. Just learning the chemical reaction and destruction drinking alcohol creates in the brain and body through oxygen depletion and the demand on the liver should make one not imbibe. We know we are destroying the body's health and reducing its function, thereby causing our life to become harder and potentially shorter. The act of smoking and the biological pandemonium it creates is a great tool for the difference of the mind and the brain organ. The brain and its functional responsibility to the body would never ask that harm be done to it. However, our learned mind and its perceived reaction to handling stress makes us go for the easy out of chemical numbing regardless of the physical damage it causes. So the mind separate from the body grabs the smoke, drink or emotionally satisfying junk food.

Therefore, it becomes only logical is to identify the source of the reaction to stress perception and practice healthful ways to deal with the reaction for the health of our temporary body. The source is always the mind. Never the brain. Of course chemical and biological imbalances through injury and illness can create damage and harm to the functions. Which only makes the case for the healthy individual to choose ways to prevent injury or illness. Yoga is the management of the distractions of the mind. If one becomes aware of the constant state of flux within the mind and its perception one can practice management of the damage the mind can inflict. Through perception of the brain as separate from the mind we can see the brains innate desire for conditions that preserve its functions and thereby the health of the body we inhabit. When the minds choices are destructive to the brain and body, leading to injury or illnesses, the body suffers. The hangover hurts because the brain tissue was damaged and needs to shut the other functions of the body down to heal the brain. So what can we do? Make better choices both in the minds perception of life's stress and its reaction to it. Or manage the mind. In doing so we create unity in the functions of the body and harmony with the events of life. However, this is not an easy undertaking.

It is a practice. So is yoga. Doctors practice that way. They own a practice. They practice at health and healing. Helping bodies recover from often times self-inflicted injury and illness. The body can turn on us and disease can create harm to the body and the doctor practices helping us heal the body because it is only temporary and if ill will cease to function. We can be the doctors of our mind and practice administering health to our brain and body within our powers. Practice managing the mind through Yoga, meditation, arts, sports, better choices. Remembering not to blame the mind when the practice becomes hard and we make poor choices is the productive way to practice. Watching our ways of behaving allows us see if we are inhabiting the mind or the body as the brain and body will never choose unhealthy options, but the mind will. The brain wishes to function optimally and wants the body to live. The mind knows the body will perish eventually. Therefore, wouldn't it make sense to want to create the environment of health and wellbeing if we want to inhabit a healthy body and sustain its life? Every breath becomes a meditation. Each heartbeat contains the creation of life. The healthy skin allows sensory experience in unique ways. Life becomes a constant gift and we practice taking care of each valuable temporary and fragile moment we are in the body. We practice healthy.

Your experience counts

Ultimately, it falls to the student to begin seeking and questioning. I could list scores of experiments that track the benefits in meditators lives. Many study groups have been formed and the results profiled. Rather than pick a favorite study to prove the benefits of meditation and have you read about someone else's experience I offer you an alternative. I encourage you to try some techniques on yourself and see if you notice any results. Search, seek and known as, Shakespeare tell us. I like to practice a new technique for thirty days in my real life situations. How does it affect my mind or body? If I notice something positive, I may work on it longer or put it in my wheel house to use as needed. Often times comparing your story to others may lead to doubt and misunderstanding. Follow your inner voice and trust where it takes you. Try out different methods of meditation and see how they work for you. Applying these principals to real life situations are the litmus test for me in my life. If I can insert the learnings and ideas from these practices in a non-yoga situation in my life and they work then I know that it is the truth, for me.

I set the intention to use my practice in real life. Any time we feel distracted in life or our yoga class, we can use a meditation, mind management or mindfulness technique in most situations without anyone knowing what we are doing. I will use the term 'total engagement concept' techniques or T.E.C. for my purposes. Once learned, these tools can be in our tool box for life. Listening to the sound of the breath, feeling the flow of the breath, focusing on the feeling of the body, the temperature of the room, the smell of our environment, the sound of music, or a spot across the room are T.E.C. techniques I use. Notice when the brain is scattered by distractions such as a noisy person, a negative conversation, ego reacting to a perceived threat, the temperature of the room or the wide variety of situations and stimuli that steal energy. Noticing, or as my teacher Amrit Desai names it, witnessing, is the first step. Our energy level determines our abilities. If we practice noticing attention flowing away and perceive it as electricity leaving a source, we will become aware of how tangible it is. After noticing the existence of our body and brains energy becoming aware of its existence we can move on to step two.

The focus technique or techniques that work, when learned through experience, become a trigger response, or habit, that brings one back to a place of balance. The list of possible T.E.C. techniques is endless and takes experimentation to find the one suitable for your situation. Observing your shift away from center and a source that is taking away energy is step one, implementing a technique is step two. The method of brining awareness into the present moment and interrupting nonproductive responses by replacing them with techniques that keep us centered and retaining energy is called mindfulness. I find that breathing exercises, or pranayama, extending the length of breath works the best for me. When noticing a distraction, I take a long breath in through my nostrils, retain the breath in my lungs and contemplate my gratefulness for something, someone, or some place. I then release the breath in a long exhale out of my nostrils and hold the breath out for a comfortable amount of time. Then rinse and repeat. This dials my mind in immediately and restores energy to my system. It is simplistic in nature and a very old technique of retaining the breath in and out but works quickly and efficiently. It can be used in the middle of an argument, in traffic, on the phone, in class and even in the middle of a store. It takes me right into myself and leads to step three.

Step three is practicing the total engagement concept technique that works for you, frequently and often. It can change over time, evolving as you do. The technique that used to work best for me was to make a hand gesture, or sacred Mudra that reminded me of meditating. Bringing the first finger and thumb together is an ancient sign of the outer world and inner world meeting together. The tiny gap between the two fingers can be representative of the consciousness of the inner and outer worlds. That technique, while instantly calming to me, does not have the same effect it uses to on me. Put many techniques into your tool box. There is no right or wrong and only experience can change one's perceptions of situations. Find the one that works for you and don't be afraid to use it.

CHAPTER NINE
Why do a yoga retreat or workshop?

"If you think you are enlightened go spend a week with your family."

-Ram Das

Ram Das says it with humor, which is one of the reasons I fell in love with his teachings first. He has not lost that touch of dry wit even through surviving and thriving with a stroke. He continues to smile when he teaches wisdom with a sly grin. When I first started to seek something deeper in life after losing my brother, his martial arts teacher gave me a set of old bootleg Ram Das talks as I previously stated. His mix of spiritual seeking, God, Jewish and Hindu beliefs mixed with humor were something I had never heard before. As is usual, his truths are surprising but undeniable. Our family can teach us so much about ourselves. What we like and dislike. So often we need to get away from our comfort zone to truly grow though. Getting outside our box can push us forward on our path. At some point, you may want to try more than just yoga classes in a group format. To get outside the yoga family you have created or to just go deeper than a class. There are many reasons for wanting to do more than just take a yoga class. The challenge lies in choosing the right workshop for you. The instructor takes much more time preparing for a workshop than a class so that it is comfortable for you and informative. A workshop can present information you hear in Yoga all the time in a new and exciting way, or it can be a related subject that spurs a new interest. Add workshops to supplement your regular practice at the studio.

Wanting to learn how to do specific postures more successfully? Being able to ask questions of the teacher and learn specifics about alignment and form at the beginning makes you a safer and better practitioner. Perhaps you would like to know more about a specific style of Yoga that is not offered regularly on the schedule or a related subject like Qigong, a workshop is an excellent way to do just that.

Are there postures you see others do or that go buy to fast in a regular class? Workshops are the time to understand the why of Yoga? Why am I doing this posture, what is it doing for me and how do I do it correctly. Being better educated about the details of these postures prevents injuries and allows you to know exactly what the purpose of the postures is. Adding in a few extra hours this month of Yoga by taking a workshop could be the challenge your body needs. Perhaps you are almost into that balancing posture the way you want but can't quite get it. Maybe you trying to get those tight hamstrings to finally loosen up a bit more or need some strength in that core. A few extra hours in a workshop this month could be just what you need physically, mentally; emotionally or spiritually to take that leap of growth you're looking for.

A workshop takes days, months, years of experience to plan and execute. By attending you get to learn from an experienced master teacher about their passions. What is it that lights them up and makes them want to give what they have received to others? Allow them to pour their knowledge, experience and passions into your practice. Take what resonates with you, practice the information, let it affect you and leave what doesn't work for you behind. Some of the instructors teach workshops just to be able to get to know you one on one and give their love of material a new life in you. Make it a Yoga party. Team up with your friends, family and partners and bring them with you for a unique bonding time at a workshop. Not only will your bond grow closer with those you already know, but you will invariably meet others who share your likes and concerns at a workshop.

Retreating far and away

Taking a retreat is a popular thing to do. Sometimes we think we need to go somewhere exotic and foreign with a director planning our every minute. India. Lots of Lingams, Yoni's, too. So many Lingams and Shiva temples, they are all really a blur at this point. I had no idea such ancient places still were accessible to people. Temples that predate recorded history, an ancient trading port with Rome, just amazing. You really feel and see the effects of time on the planet. Going to India changed my life. My ideas of what make me feel safe were destroyed and what safety means was re defined. All I could say when I was getting on the plane was to leave was I will never come here again, and now all I want to do is go back to my teacher's temple at Kiyavarohan. I would like to be in that holy spot. There was one other Ashram in Pondicherry I would like to go to again and study, but I really want to see North India which is supposed to be so different. Most of the trip, we were in the oldest part of India down south and not much has changed in eons. It was breathtaking, it really gave me a new perspective even though I was well traveled before going.

On our last day at the temple, we had a rare experience. We accompanied our teacher to the meditation house of his teacher. This was the room the master had meditated in everyday for hours when the temple was being built. The temple attendants had kept everything exactly as it had been thirty years before. We were led downstairs to a sacred chamber not open to the public. Our teacher was visibly moved as we entered the space that contained the mat laid out where the master had meditated. It felt as if the master had just left the space. It looked like he would return at any minute. Every spot was clean as it would have been when he was there. The teacher's harmonium was in the corner and his alter was still set with his gurus and teachers pictures. Our teacher was extremely reverent and led us into a deep meditative state. He led us into a few prayers and then a silent meditation. After a length of time people began to find their way outside again. When meditating I go quite deep and sometimes sit for three or four hours. It was not quite that long but I remember as I came to I and one other lady from the group were the only ones left. We silently left.

As we exited I noticed what a beautiful hot day in North Eastern India it was. Everything seemed to be lit up even though it was a bright sunny day. It was as if everything I looked at was illuminated from the inside. The sunlight and its reflection was so intense I could not look at it. The colors seemed heightened. On the walk back our teacher's son stopped to talk to a lovely older Indian lady who had lived there since the master had been there. As he spoke to her I noticed how beautiful she was. I could see the body she was in but when I looked at her it was as if I was looking at a twenty-year-old version of herself. She truly glimmered. He would speak to her in the local language and then translate what she had said. I had the sense though that while I could not understand her language, I could understand what she meant. As if I had my own translator in my head. It was the oddest feeling, but I really could understand what she was saying before it was translated.

I was silent most of the rest of the morning as I took photos and prepared to leave. As I climbed aboard the coach, I could feel my heart strings being pulled, as I would feel if I was leaving someplace significantly important to me personally, such as leaving my parents' home. I really appreciated the magnificence of the temple and had learned much on this leg of our trip. I did not know why I should feel attached to the place. My teacher came on board, and sat next to me. He had never sat this close to me before. As we began to pull away from the temple I silently thanked the master teacher and said that I would miss his home and where he spent so much time. I heard a voice in my mind that answered back clearly stating, "I am not here, I am everywhere, carry me in your heart and that is where I will be." I know that I will never look at the world the same after being in India. I am forever grateful for the person who sponsored my trip so I could have the experience. I cannot describe the experience to others well. All I find myself saying is that there are no words to describe the experience of India. If I had not gone on this Yoga retreat, my whole existence would be different on the planet. I discovered the magic of a retreat from all of life and day to day perspectives that get stuck. I vowed then to go on retreats throughout life to come.

When choosing a retreat, a student should investigate the retreat history, host and the good and not so good of the locale. There were times in India where I actually feared for my life. One time in particular when my bicycle taxi driver was mobbed and beaten will stay with me forever. It was in an alley in a sacred place in southern India and the only way I feel I survived was through the level head that meditation has created for me to access. A student should get the itinerary beforehand and know the scheduled stops and be prepared for unscheduled stops. The world has changed a lot in many places in the last decade since I went to India. Once should consider the political and social climes of the local. A Boy Scout is prepared has served me well all these years. Thanks to a friend preparing with natural medicines, herbs and flowers, the one time I contracted an unsettled stomach it did not last long and I was spared a serious disorder. Make sure when researching your first retreat, especially if it is international, that you know everything you can know about your group, its leader and the local.

Retreating closer to home

I recently returned from my version of a mini retreat. I knew I just needed a serious break and wanted to feel supported and loved. I have several friends in Florida and my Yoga teacher's school is there. My Guru, Yogi Amrit Desai, was offering a few shorter trainings I thought would be supportive and relaxing and a friend had invited me to stay with her right on the water the week before they began so I stayed at the beach with my sweet friend for the first week. I didn't remember what it was like waking up to the sound of birds instead of an alarm. I left the beach for the old growth, thousands year old forest where the Amrit Institute is located. I found out I had to rent a car at the last minute which could have been very stressful. But my friend supported me and made sure I was off safely. When I got my room assignment I was to stay in the Guru's house. I was lit up. I saw a CD pile laying at check in and asked about it, feeling like I should but didn't want to ask for any favors. I was told they had been giving them out and there was just a few left. I put it in my bag with gratitude and settled in my room. Yoga Nidra was at five.

There are some places we remember forever. The smell, the feeling, the air quality, is all imprinted in our memory. The Darshan (practice) room at the Institute is permanently a part of the recesses of my being. So much transformation, revelations, awakening, emotional catharsis has happened there, and I'm just talking about me personally. Entering there for the first time in years is like reentering the womb. I allowed myself to just receive on this retreat. That night I debated about listening to the CD they gave out at check in. Finally, I slipped on the headphones. My ears are filled with the sweet voice of my Guru's daughter, Kamini. The words entrance me. It's like someone is pulling on a thread tied to something vaguely familiar. As she speaks about stepping into your presence a lightning storm explodes in my mind. I was there. I know those words she is speaking. My mind lights up in a 3d scene. I am again sitting in the room where this was recorded. Her words pierce my heart. Then a tsunami of feelings engulfs my every fiber of being. I hear my voice speaking. It's trembling, filed with emotions. That day was the birth of my new life as a Yogi, as my Guru's life student. That day was a precipice in my life and I hear it in my voice on the recording. Then I remember further back to my first graduation from Yoga Nidra training. I left it seeing the world through foreign eyes. I would never be the same from that day forward. I feel a vacuum as if I traveled at the speed of light and am sucked back into the present moment, sitting on the bed with the headphones on. I can't believe where I've come from to where I am now on my path as a Yogi. I have such a simpler approach to the world and its ups and downs. I have practiced the witness perspective and non-reactive lessons they teach at Amrit. My whole way of being in the world changed since those first trainings and that recording. My heart swells with gratefulness. You never know how far you've come until you go back. We think we're deciding to be at a certain place at a certain time never knowing that we are being placed there for a reason. We think someone is randomly giving us a

CD to listen to when actually it is divine intervention. The rest of the weekend was a blur of hearing my Guru's familiar teachings and friendly participants. I was really in shock.

We should trust the sages in our lives. Reside in the heart; there is nowhere else to be. If we reside fully in our Hara (heart center) and fill the recesses with light, there is nowhere for darkness, guilt, shame, doubt and fear to hide. Back in Orlando I got to see my first meditation teacher Diane Ross. To me she is the definition of the word ethereal. I am bonded to her in ways only my soul knows. She is the wise guide I needed to manifest so long ago who I can't imagine not having met. After suffering the tragic loss of my brother to a motorcycle accident I ran away to Florida. I was at a pinnacle in my life where I faced a turning point. I could easily have traveled down the path one of my friends took. The one of darkness, drugs and late night binges. Or I could listen to the voice in my head commanding me to go to meditation with Diane. I listened to that command and have been her student all these years. I met her in her new office still fresh from the Ashram, this time around, and I had a very powerful and transformative meditation with her that was too intensely personal and revelatory for me to share all of here. Fueled by my experience at the Ashram, having been the witness to the full circle of my life, hearing the voice of my old and shaky voice on that recording, my session with Diane permanently placed my soul in residence in my heart center. I'll never be the same. I love her. I love myself. My heart is filled with light. The next week with my best friend was in fast forward. I have known her since college when she smiled at me in the book store so many years ago and we have been in each other's lives since. With her I get to lay down my serious side and be my silly self. We saw movies and the new Harry Potter attraction at Universal Studios, ate bad food and stayed up late.

Holding hands and having a best friend is better than theme parks and equal to having a Guru. I have been blessed with many true and loving friends in all my travels. Three have been lifelong friends through it all. Debbie, Dorothy and Eric have been there through the ups and downs. From these friends I have received strength, love, support and continuity. I have learned from them. A Guru teaches us. We learn from them, consistently.

I returned to the Ashram in the Florida forest for a scripture study weekend. I was reunited with sweet souls I had not seen in years. It was reaffirmed that I have a home there, an extended family. I was confirmed in my being that I am a Yogi. The knowledge my Guru shared is too vast to divulge here but hearing him answer my questions about the Bhagavad Gita and the character Arjuna not wanting to kill his own family will forever resonate within me and those present. When agendas are no longer useful people can love more. Find a living master and just love them. After about three days of acclimating to being on a retreat or in the ashram setting I notice that people really relax in a way I have never seen. It is so profoundly altering that people's very faces shape shift. Once the phones are off and the computer is off and a schedule where food is provided at the same time each day and Yoga and meditation are programmed, a change happens. It is what I base my Yoga studio, Sun Salute Yoga on. In a safe environment, where we feel protected and provided for, we lose the need of a hidden agenda and a true transformation can and will occur. This type of learning could not have happened in the comfort of home, surrounded by the familiarity of family. I had to go outside my box to have an eye opening experience.

Leading a retreat to Bali was also one of the most educational experiences I have had in yoga and life. Learning to trust a guide and follow them into unchartered waters is a big commitment to make. Observing what creates reactions in ourselves and others can be so enlightening. In Bali there are snakes hanging from trees, a particular phobia of mine, rain and water, monkeys that steal and throw, beaches hidden in forest that only locals no how to find and the rooms only have half walls and not windows allowing anything to enter at any time of the night. In India, my friend Scott and I used to practice finding our edges, going outside our comfort zones and seeing how far off the beaten or known path we could go. Elizabeth Gilberts Eat Love Pray book is filled with the lessons she learned from her retreat around the world and has inspired countless people to strike out on their own adventures. We grow through challenges and the unexpected. The key is as Amrit Desai says to not get edgy on the edge. Can you grow and learn about yourself in these foreign situations? Place yourself in these situations, either in a workshop on a subject outside of your box, or a faraway land on retreat and see how you grow.

I love Japanese food. Moving from California to Japan as a little seven-year-old was a huge culture shock. I looked everywhere for a hardboiled egg only to find raw ones that you stir in steaming hot rice to create scrambled eggs in rice. The deserts made into fantastical art work stand out in my memory and I never saw anything like them until traveling to Paris as an adult. Buddhist temples with brilliant colored silk and great ringing bells amazed me with wide eyed wonder as a little boy. Women in fanciful traditional dress patting my blonde curls with their beautiful brown skin and then giggling charm my memories. Because I was on this four-year retreat as a little boy, I was forced outside comfort zones, taught that everything foreign is entrancing rather than frightening and learned so much about the wonder of the world and its cultures and diversity. This young experience has colored my life and kept me on a constant quest for the new and learning experiences offered by being outside our box. I encourage you, in yoga or life to take on learning with a joy of life and expand in all directions at all times.

CHAPTER TEN
Why to NOT do yoga?

"What is right is not always popular and what is popular is not always right."   **- Albert Einstein**

I do not tell people that I do yoga, nor do I call myself a yogi anymore. Having learned meditation a decade before being introduced to yoga, I have always felt more like a meditator that was studying yoga. I approached learning yoga like I do everything else. I realized it was a passion of mine so I jumped in with both feet. The yoga I do now has nothing to do with the yoga that is popular today. My friends know that I never subscribe to what is popular. I am such a history buff and love to know what has survived as timeless over the ages. I meditated a decade before learning yoga. Then after three years into yoga I found my teacher with a sixty-year history of teaching yoga. He learned yoga growing up in India from his teacher. I studied with him and his teachers for six years before I began exploring my own practice of yoga. I believe that one should feel empowered to, at some point, take what they have learned and adapt it into their own practice or needs. That is why there are, at the current popularity rate of yoga, literally thousands upon thousands of different forms of yoga out there. I personally find it all a bit confusing and potentially damaging as well as helpful in introducing new students to yoga. Yoga today shows up in such a multitude of forms. Every year a new slew of super star yoga teachers leads trainings and retreats around the globe. There is an agency, booking, sponsorship, marketing system in place just like any professional athletic sport in the world. There is even a movement to get yoga into the Olympics. I don't know or have anything to do with this version of yoga. I don't teach at festivals, I have led retreats and teacher trainings, I have meditated over twenty years and now studied yoga for twelve but I am not a pop yogi.

In the pop yoga world, you will find everything from yoga for abs, butt, thighs, and combined with the latest exercise trends from ballet to carnival tricks. You can also go the other route and attend spiritual combo events led by dreadlock beheaded pseudo hippies wearing Indian themed sarongs that spout a dialog of spiritual soup, that combines every major religion into a love poem that makes everyone feel good. What I am suggesting is that you as the student take the time to ask why you are there. What does what is being presented to you have to do with yoga? How is it helping you? What benefits are you receiving? And just to make me happy, is it going to prevent injury? Is it in alignment with your ethics? Are there reasons not to be doing yoga?

Having meditated for ten years before being introduced into yoga gave me a unique perspective on the ancient discipline of yoga. I very much see yoga as a martial art. It should garner the same lengthy and rigorous dedication as learning the art of self-defense. I am outspoken in the belief that I think yoga should be regulated. I like to follow the rules and standards set before us for our good and the good of society. Our hair stylist is heavily regulated and it is required that they have continuing education to retain their license. They are more regulated than the people teaching yoga. I became a personal trainer first but had been a health and exercise nut for twenty years previously. I took nine personal training courses over the beginning years of my career. Knowing the anatomy and what was safe and dangerous practice was my primary interest. I wanted to subscribe to the idea that exercise needed to be individualized for the client. This is the philosophy behind my yoga teaching as well.

The student should be coached individually to meet them where they are on their path. In my world the teacher should know about the student's physical limitations, injuries and match their growth at their path. Most yoga is taught in a busy and filled yoga class room where individual attention is rare. In the individual growth method of teaching and learning, new information or knowledge was only given by the teacher when the student was ready. The student would have to study with the teacher for many years to learn the ins and outs of the teachings. A student may have to practice and live a posture and philosophy for up to a year before progressing onto the next lesson. However, that is not how yoga is disseminated in today's world. There are no regulations and anything can be labeled yoga by anyone who wants to pick up the mantle of yoga.

In what is called yoga now, students are bombarded with a mixologist special of inspiring quotes, vague spiritual direction from all religions are espoused, postures are invented, yoga teachers steal clients from studios and start their own classes, a wide variety of scandals are swept under the rug and safety is nary mentioned. As a studio owner and teacher I already knew many studio owners before I opened my doors. I believe what made me such a successful teacher is that I followed the moral code of yoga. When I was at a studio I only talked about that studio to the students there. When asked if I taught anywhere else I would only acknowledge when I was at that studio teaching. Staying friends with those other studio owners as I became one myself was something I prided myself on. I acted in such a respectable way that these other business owners, could have seen my opening a studio as a threat.

Morals and Ethics

Through them and others I have heard so many stories of intrigue and stealthy behaviors from both studio owners and yoga teachers. Recently I heard from a teacher in California who partnered with two other teachers to open a studio. Within two years the other two teachers became a romantic couple. They then decided to push her out and she opened her own studio not very far from the original location. Many of the students followed her to her new studio but she lost her original investment. This is just one of many stories I have heard of impropriety in the yoga world. These stories do not surprise me anymore. One impropriety that seems harmless on the surface is donation yoga. Sold as free, at first it seems noble. According to law, the studios legally operate as if they were a nonprofit entity. A donation based, for profit business, flown under the guise of community service. The law clearly states that only a nonprofit can accept donations as its main source of income. The studio independent contractors are actually employees therefore breaking the law as an employer and not paying unemployment insurance or property taxes. In the name of yoga, illegal business is allowed to flourish while tax paying and law abiding businesses are going out of business by trying to follow the law? Is the yoga you are thinking of trying following a moral code or is it a reason to not do yoga?

The point of this chapter is not to dissuade you but to inform you and empower you. It's not that I don't want you to do yoga. I want students to look deeper than the surface. Recently I took a private client who had been a dancer and gymnast who found yoga. She really took to yoga and thought like everyone else that she was doing a great thing for her body. Little did she know, until her shoulder complex would give out after five years, that she was doing a common but extremely complicated yoga pushup and tore her rotator cuff muscle group. A tear that is common amongst athletes who respectively perform the same action incorrectly. This injury can lead to years of physical therapy and an imbalance in muscle function. Is the teacher you are going to take mindful of anatomy and the possible damage that postures done incorrectly can do to the body or are they doing damage and offering another reason not to do yoga?

Injuries due to yoga done incorrectly are more common than one would suspect. Just like other sport activities, actions, if done wrong can lead to serious problems, injury and eventually a student leaving yoga. If instructed by a qualified and well trained facilitator, students can be safe and free of injury. Learning from a qualified yoga teacher and choosing a class appropriate for your level will ensure you remain injury-free. One day I went looking for a popular hot yoga teacher. I wanted to learn more about the, at that time, new form of hot yoga. It had just come out as the latest version of Birkram Yoga. Now people were teaching and taking hot yoga classes mixed with traditional power yoga methods. So as I went looking for this popular teacher, I found that his name was no longer on the studios class list. It appeared that he did not teach any classes that week. I went to the studio and asked the front desk staff if he was on a break. The lady working at the front counter looked at me with a grimace and said "Um, He no longer works here." I found out he had been let go for dating a student who was of the age of 16. The lesson of which is that it is very important to check things out before just following along with what is popular.

As has come to light, even the founder of the method of hot yoga has come under fire for alleged misappropriate conduct. The path of yoga in America is not easy and one can find many reasons not to do yoga. There are multitudes of stories of all kinds. I am not condoning negative thinking. It is important to focus on all the good that yoga is doing and why people from all walks of life are doing or teaching yoga. However, it is wise to be educated and to know one's risks in starting any new adventure. I was following a popular yoga teacher who led his practice from the heart. He had a great way of teaching postures. He would start you out in a simple pose but through his manner of coaxing his students into small short held poses he would eventually lead to very complex poses. I loved his teaching style. It was all heart-based, but the practice was challenging. We would wind up on some really difficult to teach poses but without knowing we were going there. It was opposite of my style of teaching which I liked. I have always loved exploring the what is the opposite of my perspective, on subjects. He was so good I signed up for a weekend retreat in Los Angeles and looked forward to meeting him in person.

The class was mind blowing good. I had no idea with my neck and knee concerns that I could get into some of those postures. But his method of teaching was surprisingly effective. The room was wall to wall or mat to mat. People were in all different stages of the poses, but similar, according to bodily limitations. We were sweating and groaning and panting at times. The teacher's voice was over a microphone and was seductively leading us through strange places with our bodies. It was an intoxicating experience. It was similar to my guru's style of teaching, but with much more instructing and more challenging postures. The atmosphere was very casual after the workshop classes. Everyone seemed to be in a dream like state and the teacher was in the lobby just greeting people as they came by. I approached and introduced myself. Just being in his presence, I recognized a charge of energy similar to my guru's energy field. It was a masculine energy, stronger than my teachers but kind. I could tell he was a good guy but something felt withheld. I enjoyed talking to him and thanked him for his teaching's. We spoke until a very attractive lady walked up.

It was not long after that I heard some controversy around his business dealings. Several official emails were released on both sides of the story and it all seemed so intensely private. I was wondering why so much private material was being discussed publicly. I did not see how any personal dealings should be made public. I could not connect how his private affairs would have influenced his teachings. I had never heard him speak while teaching about the Yama's and Niyama. He spoke a lot about the heart and love and compassions. I never considered his morals as relevant to his yoga teachings. I was not holding the teacher up on a pedestal of perfections. I heard he slept with his financier who was married at the time. After the scandal broke he moved to Mexico and left behind his yoga empire of heart based yoga. Many of his teachers quit calling themselves teachers of his style and a new group was formed to run his trainings and company. Did he create a fantastic heart based style of yoga or was he creating another reason not to do yoga?

Even my teacher was accused of some controversy more than twenty years ago. He never left his yoga path though. If anything the unfounded accusations that never proceeded past rumors drove him further into his own personal practice. He had created the largest yoga center in America and had to leave it all behind with his loyal family in tow. Everything he created from nothing as an immigrant was lost on the basis of accusations from those that stood to gain everything he had built for nothing. He gave up his life's mission of bringing a traditional based yoga to the west in the name of his guru who had given him everything. Rather than face a costly legal battle over finger pointing, he gave it all away as a yoga would do. He retreated into seclusion. Having all the energy that he had been spending outside of himself running the largest yoga facility in America returned to him and allowed him to spend this energy on his own practice. He could have gone into dark depression and regret and became consumed with loathing for those he had trusted the most. Instead he went deep inside and retreated from civil duties for deep seclusion. He was only coaxed out to teach again by his own personal calling and the requests of students. His teachings are brilliant and insightful and cut through all the dogma of most yoga practices. He takes students straight to the source and his messages are clear and unclouded. When I first starting following his teachings, he was delivering a lot of Shaktipat energy every time he taught.

At the time I did not know about this yogic power that advanced yogis can access. Shakti is defined in 'Prana and Pranayama by Sarasvati' as: "Primal energy; manifest consciousness; subtle creative and vital energy." Usually shaktipat is considered a transferring of energy from the teacher to the student. However, my view of the experience is that the teacher just holds the space for the students to release our own built up or blocked energy. I don't think the energy is coming from the teacher. From my perspective, the teacher or Guru is just holding a safe space that allows energy to spontaneously speed up and release or clean some of the individual students blocks. These blocks can be perceived as karma, neurological stress and hypertension, depression, loss of health, an out of date belief, or any limiting behavior that the student may be challenged with. The body can speed up in this safe zone and work rapidly through its limitations. The experience can be frightening and maddening, or beautiful and serene. It truly depends on the perspective of the student. One usually leaves the experience with a new perspective on life.

One afternoon session in particular took me somewhere I never knew existed. We had our usual morning satsang, or speaking session, with Amrit. But at the conclusion he lingered in lotus on his chair. He began to sing a chant I had never heard. Judging by his deep vocal tone, I notice voices first, he was in his own deep meditative state. I had the knowing that this was a sacred guru mantra. a song or chant given to the disciple by their own personal guru. In this instance, that guru mantra would have come from his teacher.   I had a strong affinity for my teacher's teacher but only knew him from his pictures, as I had not started to study his teaching yet. Usually we would all stand at the end of my guru's talk and wish him well as he left. Then a funny thing happened. The whole ceiling opened up to the sky and a lightning storm replaced the ceiling. And a lightning bolt would shoot pass me and hit someone and they would start laughing about nothing, then another lightning bolt would shoot past me and hit someone and they would begin crying. Some people like him main disciple stayed calm and took the energy. But when it hit me, it hit the tip of my tailbone and rushed up to my skull. The energy built up and hit me like a volcano. I thought my head was going to explode. I was in this alternative reality where I was pure energy and could feel the energy pulsing up to my skull and wanting to exit but it couldn't.

Finally, the guru stopped chanting and he got up but most of us could not get up to give him good wishes. We were lying on the floor. It took me a long time to get back into my body. I gathered my strength and dragged myself to a bench outside and I was in an alternative universe. Everything was illuminated from within, and yet the pressure was built up so tightly at the base of the skull. I told a disciple that I wanted to take my head off like Ganesha. They suggested that I not take my head off but go wade in the water. It seemed to ground me back into my body and I went back in my room and meditated. I returned home to my life in California. One day about two weeks later, I stopped to get gas and someone looked at me and we had a connection. Then and there, I entered another way of seeing life force. Everything was light at the gas station. I had to call someone from the ashram. They explained to me what shaktipat was. This was the first I heard of it. They talked me down so I could drive home. I researched and studied the idea that a learned teacher can open up a channel for students who are ready to expedite their learning process. In all ancient texts you can find warnings that this intense opening of energy is not for everyone. It can lead to misconceptions about one's psychic abilities or amplify ones mental, physical or emotional challenges. Seeking out a true and advanced yoga master is not for everyone. Many students are not ready or have not prepared themselves through diligence and discipline to handle being propelled along their path. I make a joke about the student using a tooth brush to achieve their enlightenment. Did he abuse his powers when he was forced out of his organization years before and create a reason not to do yoga, or was he a yogi in the true sense?

Zen Buddhism is known for its disciplinary nature. Learning to dismantle one's own ego is not for the faint of heart. It takes great patience and understanding along with dedication and vision. One Zen student told a story of how his practice every day involved cleaning the bathroom at the ashram with a toothbrush as his only tool. As you can imagine it would take hours and hours of back breaking work to clean a large public bathroom this way. Through the agonizing work, one would have to certainly surrender their ego and patience. This would not be for the faint of heart or the half serious seeker. The lesson gained from the tedium of working this way to clean, especially knowing that much faster and accelerated means exist to getting the job done would be challenging for most all. However, the faster way would not gain the student patience and less ego. Therefore, quicker is not best nor for everyone. You have to use a toothbrush to achieve enlightenment. The faster way could cause many complications if the student had not done the hours of scrubbing first. Some texts even state that expedited awakening can cause symptoms of insanity. Is seeking out a master to teach a student the secrets of yoga a reason not to do yoga?

Ever since that awakening moment in my teacher's presence, I seem to be able to switch back and forth from seeing life from a meditative perspective to being more reality based. Feeling more aware of energy, how it moves through animals, plants, and through our choices, we can leave a surplus of positive energy behind, or a negative depletion of energy. Everything we decide to do, think, feel how we act and our deeds determine if we are leaving behind a surplus of energy for this planet, or a negative debt. I have been able to access this deep state of meditative awareness at will. However, it is hard to translate, let alone relate. I find it has brought me challenges in life. I see clearly and sometimes would choose not to see, yet it is there. I have learned to honor and be grateful. Even when the lessons are challenging. For me, even though at the time and subsequent months until I learned what had happened, this experience was confusing and complex. It could have easily been a reason not to do yoga.

When a fellow yoga teacher rudely explained to me that I could not follow my guru because there had been some controversy twenty years earlier, I was able to respond with repose. I appreciate my guru because he went through a literal hell, losing everything he had dedicated his life to. He kept true the only constant in his life. His yoga teaching, His family stuck by his side and stayed loyal to him. A handful of the bravest disciples went with him or came back after a few years. And he stayed true to his practice. His personal practice, growth and understanding accelerated. He grew in innumerable ways both as a man in a body and as a teacher. He was asked to teach again and when he did he was able to have a direct path to knowledge and information. In India he could see the secret yoga messages in cave paintings and sculptures. He was more devoted to the path than ever. He had grown and was sharing all he had to give.

Yogi Amrit Desai came to my studio for 'The Urge to Merge' workshop, a day of bliss. As I sat and looked at his photo I always have displayed, and looked over to the right where he was sitting, I was tickled with bliss. My Guru, who has illuminated my life, and whose words and teachings take me to the light of the Lord, was here. Full circle. Four years ago, I did not know I could grin from ear to hear. I was still lost in the missing parts. But now I feel whole again. I watched as others would laugh out loud at Gurudev's mix of insight and humor (oh God, let all my Gurus have a sense of humor). I was thrilled to see others taking notes, hearing the truth in the message. I delighted when others eyes glimpsed over at me and twinkled.

I floated on a cloud I thought was a cushion under me as I looked up at my teacher. No saint, but a man. A man who has suffered life's ups and downs, and stayed in the light of love. My heart burst at the seams, knowing this is possible for all. This is what life was about. I was so proud he was in the Yoga studio and that his teachings allowed me to create. He was in my alter to truth, light and love that I offer up to the world. I glided out the door as the day wound down and hugged him goodbye in the rain. I bravely said, 'I love you Gurudev'. My light exploded in ecstasy as he said 'I love you too,' back to me. Oh God, thank you for your teachers, Oh God, thank you for my brother, Oh God thank you for showing me the light of your love. Satnam; Truth is we are meant to live a life of light and love. Oft' times, we need to be reminded and sometimes those reminders are hard to survive, but survive we must, to shine on.

If I had not been true to myself I could have left the path at the beginning from fear rumors had created or judgement. However, I knew what my heart was saying which was to see the truth for me and follow that path. I share this with you to encourage you to look at both sides of the coin when you encounter any information. See what feels like the truth to you and follow that. Don't just jump on the gossip bandwagon, but be educated and make the right fit for you. There is something out there for all types in modern yoga. Be an investigator and look at all the reason for doing yoga and compare them to those not to do yoga. For me, the biggest concern and what comes first in every situation is safety first.

Safety First

I have always been on the side of safety first. It is probably my role as older brother. I am always trying to take care of others. I want to do whatever I can to create no friction around others. I always try my best to look out for others needs first. I guess it comes with always checking to see if my little brother Todd was safe and ok. I just didn't want to be responsible for another person getting hurt in any way. And Todd did not make it easy. He broke his arm trying to fly like Superman. One day on the swings in front of me, he sliced open his back thigh on some bolts. There was blood everywhere. What interested me is that he did not notice right away. He took several steps as he would normally. I drew his attention to the blood running down his leg and he was shocked to look down and see a huge gaping wound. Then he fell down and couldn't walk. I ran for help.

In both instances we were able to save his respective limb. Another time he and I decided to try to ride the old horse that had been put out to pasture on the neighbor's field. We were not aware at the time that we could technically be shot for trespassing on the farmer's field. I decided I was to go first and Todd would keep the horse calm. As we approached, I could feel the energy of this massive beast. So much different than a cow's energy. Todd approached the tired, old and overweight retired swayback horse. I approached from the side and when it seemed right, tried to swing myself onboard. The horse upon feeling my touch, began to buck and jump and whiney. I fell off, of course, and looked up to see my brother long gone. Then it dawned on me that he could have been trampled and hurt so I took off running after.

We both came out shaken, but ok from the farm horse incident. We keep up our rag tag ways most days, roaming around the creeks of Kansas, Missouri and Iowa. But I've always taken the older brother role with most people. I watch out for most people's safety and wellbeing. Having that nature helped me in the giving role of teaching others yoga. I care about their bodies' health and wellbeing above a hot looking showoff posture. Injuring yourself in vain is not worth it. After having my own biking accident in Scotland I really began to value slowing down a bit from my hot yoga, power yoga obsessions. But I just had perfected my headstand before the wreck. I had a deep spiritual experience while on the pavement that is very personal to me. Luckily I was wearing a helmet that literally as the doctor pointed out, saved my life.

After some minor plastic surgery, I realized that I could have suffered severe whiplash and felt as though I might not be able to perform my yoga practice. I was not ready to give up my hard earned posture practice. After my physical therapy I still couldn't take yoga but I was able to teach. I really learned a lot about how it instructs postures without having to do the postures as my neck would not allow me to do much. I still remember crying onetime while teaching a class because I thought I might never be able to do even the basic poses. Once I got stronger, I began as a student again. The only place my neck would allow me to enter was gentle yoga. I had to learn to slow way down and consider being able to hold postures much longer. Iyengar was a really personal hell for me.

The class was the slowest yoga I had ever taken. There were no fancy postures. We would spend an hour and half on the most basic of moves. We used all types of props and ropes and things I had never seen in a class. I remember once walking out of an Iyengar class years before when the teacher got out folding chairs. I was thankful this teacher did not have those folding chairs of pain. The Iyengar yoga class led to just gentle yoga classes. At least they moved a little more and they did more postures and there was music. But the pace was pretty much a death march. So slow I really had to use my meditation skills to not run from the room.

I am still recovering from the neck injury and have grown a lot both spiritually and physically. The doctors advised me to never do a headstand again, which is so challenging because I love doing headstands. However, nothing is worth risking injury again. Recently I had the worse flair up in six hears. I woke up one morning after my nightly stretch unable to put my head back on literally. My skull was dramatically off the right, which is the side of my injury. I had pulled something along my spine doing a dip. The pain was exquisite. It took eight weeks of the most intense constant pain I have ever felt. I could not function at work and my mood was complete exasperation. I can really relate to injury and limitations and the pain and suffering they can cause. Over the course of my teaching career I have had all types of students with injuries come to yoga to find a fix or remedy. Some have been recommended by their doctors, some have come from other popular exercise fads and some have even come from other yoga classes and teachers where they have suffered serious injuries. I could have let my injuries be a reason not to do yoga or a reason to explore other yoga options for healing and therapy.

"Yoga is not exercise. If you think it is, you have never been to exercise."- Golssa Moridi   I agree with Glossa's quote. When treated simply like an exercise, even with qualified instructors, yoga can be damaging and destructive. As I mentioned before in the book, even former athletes can suffer injuries in a poorly taught,

competitive and crowded studio environment. According to the U.S. Department of Health and Human Services, Public Health Service, Centers for Disease Control and Prevention, National Center for Chronic Disease Prevention and Health Promotion, Division of Nutrition and Physical Activity. Promoting physical activity: a guide for community action. Champaign, IL: Human Kinetics, 1999, yoga makes the moderate exercise list. Designed to measure energy in units called MET's. One MET is equivalent to sitting quietly for an adult. Somewhere between three and six MET's is where Yoga falls. While yoga improves us in many areas that are well documented and the benefits are great, it should not be viewed or treated as exercise, even though that is how it is popularly seen in the West. Is poorly adapted yoga exercise that can cause sports injury by repeating actions incorrectly a reason not to do yoga or does it provide some benefits?

Training Counts

Teachers are pumped out in a weekend intro training course and set loose on unsuspecting students. Once in a crowded and popular class it is easy to get lost and is impossible for a teacher to intimately work with each student to avoid injury. Although it legally does not protect the teacher and studio from lawsuits, most teachers have the students sign a liability waiver before beginning class because of the risk of injury. Teachers who are trying to make their class the hardest and most complex class can't make adjustments for all the limitations that their students may have. Especially if the student does not know or feel empowered to tell the teacher what they may be dealing with. I have been to popular classes where the teacher had no idea what they were teaching or physically asking their students to do and the injury it was going to create over time.

Sometimes the classes are taught in 116-degree heat, to loud rock music and filled with everyone from teens to midlife students who are receiving no instruction as the teacher is performing along with them.

It is not worth it to risk your health and injury and create a reason not to do yoga. The student should be extremely picky in who they decide to follow and not just follow the crowd or cheapest buck into a dangerous situation. I have had students come in from cross training boot camp fitness classes with torn hamstrings, damaged biceps and shoulders who forced themselves to do 120 repetitions of some military exercise. People have come to me after doing 20 or thirty minutes of repetitive squats on point like a ballet student at the bar who had never been to a ballet class their whole lives and are unable to even walk after. Near me there was a popular park yoga class that would attract hundreds of students from children to grannies. I would always get students who had been and hurt themselves trying to keep up with the headstands and back bends that the twenty-year-old teacher was incorrectly guiding them through. I was so thankful that I was a personal trainer before I became a yoga instructor so that I could have a greater understanding of the body and keeping safety in mind, instead of creating a reason not to do yoga.

While yoga can count as a strengthening and balancing improving activity, it is not cardio and was never intended to fit into a breakneck fast pace exercise. There is well documented proof that yoga can increase balance, flexibility, strength, lower blood pressure, help with post-traumatic stress, and create a calm approach to life, if taught correctly, methodically and with care in an intimidate and safe environment. Other than avoiding the trendy, packed room of yoga for rock hard abs and preventing injury, feel empowered to say no. Just like I did to the celebrity Los Angles teacher when she mocked me in front of 200 peers at a workshop in Laguna Niguel for not straightening my arms for over two minutes (I counted) while holding them over head. She did not take the time to find out if I had a limitation or injury. She proceeded to acclaim that this was an advanced class and perhaps I should have chosen a different class. This is a teacher that came from Los Angles that is followed by thousands and teaches a teacher training program that she invented. For me, she is creating a reason not to do yoga even though so many love her. Feel empowered to not do what they or everyone else is suggesting if it does not feel safe. Satisfying someone else's or my ego by risk of my health and wellbeing is not worth it. Knowing your bodies limitations and not doing what a teacher is bullying the other students into doing is a powerful place to be and takes courage to say no.

Ethics, safety and finally moral considerations are all reasons NOT to do yoga. What mores are important to you to expose yourself to? Why are you doing yoga? What are you hoping to get out of it? Why are you there on your mat? If the teacher, class, environment, ethics, morals, safety are not in alignment with your personal premise, why are you there? Don't get me wrong. All one has to do is open a popular yoga magazine and they can see ads for the latest new designer outfit, stylishly redesigned yoga mat touted by a celebrity or be enticed to some far off retreat or festival where a catchy named D.J. plays trance and a shaman from Peru introduces students the magic of jungle psychedelics.

When I started to teach I was really familiar with the anatomy of the body and meditation. However, having just completed my training, I have to admit I was probably a terrible yoga teacher. As I stated earlier, I just did the class with the students at the front of the room. I was actually doing yoga, not teaching yoga or being yoga. Looking back, I am surprised how full my classes were. I kept it all about the anatomy and the physical benefits of yoga and ways to stay calm through meditation techniques in the harder postures. We flowed, raised our heart rate and sweated. Yoga with weights, cardio yoga, core yoga, I did as many styles of fitness yoga that I could think of. I wore the yoga clothes I saw the other guys wear in the magazine and read Yoga Journal faithfully. I incorporated the latest trends in exercise, went to conventions where I paid top dollar to take classes from the yogis I saw in DVD and ads. I traveled to Los Angeles and New York to learn what I thought was yoga. Every month someone was creating a new type of yoga and I wanted to learn it all. I was not teaching yoga. I might have even been creating reasons not to do yoga.

Can you look at the way your teacher is leading their life and tell that they are living and breathing yoga? Is your teacher so busy that they forget to apply the principals that they were preaching to their own life? Being of the world but not in the world can be very confusing for us and for those learning from us. I have struggled with many of the Yoga dictates myself. I often go back and forth between austerity and indulgence. Most people would call me a tantric yogi. Though it is not the path of my teacher's teacher, I think as most find out that it takes that thing called balance to get by. If we spend all our time in meditation, we cannot function in the real world. If we indulge in the distractions of the worldly ways to excess, we cannot retreat to a cave to meditate. It is a fine line. You have to find what works for you. My belief is very Tantric. Life is to be lived and in it is the learning lessons we need, but our quality of life is immensely improved when we apply the knowledge of the art of Yoga and the lessons we learn are of greater value. The best place to start improving is the physical, the body. Because of that I understand the modern craze of just looking at yoga as an exercise. I also see the risk in this.

Yoga teachers should bring together all systems of the being and provide a holistic experience to their students. Understanding the muscular, skeletal, neurological, emotional, mental, intellectual and 'other' and correlating how they all function in unison, one effecting the other will give a well-rounded perspective of the multi layered experience students can have. Each student is having their own experience in any given moment in each posture. They all have their own 'why' that they showed up on the mat in your class that day, at that hour, and are having a unique moment. Their 'why' may be purely physical and they want to know how the posture is helping their body. On another hand, they may be seeking emotional solace as their motivator and knowing that a heart opening posture will help them release old emotions may be what they hear. Your instructions and guidance will be so much richer and well-rounded and you will affect others in ways they may not have known possible if you can be a dynamic, informed and conscious facilitator.

Why?

The reason why we all are showing up is individual to each of us. Why are you here, doing this at this moment? What is your personal meaning? Dedicate your practice to that why. It will never be wrong. The immediate answer you get when you close your eyes and ask yourself this simple question, is your truth. The next moment, when a thought, usually a doubt, fear or reaction, it is the mind, rational and reasoning that is speaking. The first answer you get is the true reason you are wherever you are in that exact moment. That is the lesson. This simple question, forces the mind and body out of the way and creates a direct path to your personal truth. Stay in that moment. Even when just starting to try yoga, or if you have been dedicated for years.

Once you have your clarity, notice your reaction to it. Then dedicate your thoughts, actions, words and deeds to that answer. This has helped me immensely in the energy I spend on others drama in life. My usual answer to the announcement of drama from another person is to simply allow it to happen. I refuse to be taken to wherever the other person is and dealing with life from their perspective. I used to be taken to anger when encountering someone who was dealing with anger. I would meet them where they are. But I have learned that all that does is alienate and drain me of my energy. So I try to react to the dramas of life by not reacting. 'Ok' or 'I understand' is usually all I give back to confrontation. It is easier to move on and accept their truth than fight back or try to change. I am not in charge of their life's choices. As a friend, Colby told me once; 'When someone shows you who they are, believe it.'. I believe it and do the best to remove myself from the situation because I recognize that this is their life's work and that they will recreate the exact same relationship with someone else. I am working on not repeating mistakes in this life so find it easier to move on than expend energy on something unfixable.

"A Warrior of the Light listens to what his opponent has to say. He only fights if absolutely necessary." Warrior of the Light; Paulo Coelho

I always have my student stop, close their eyes and ask themselves 'Why am I here in this moment? Why am I here and what do I hope to get out of it?" These questions guide my life. I encourage you to approach the art of yoga with clarity and understanding. It is vast, unique in its unification, but individual in its results. I encourage you to ask yourself this question before trying yoga. If you are a veteran, I invite you to ask yourself the why of your doing. Are you doing this posture in this sequence for this reason that you have been doing but not questioning its why? If not questioning one's individual why, at least question what the group is doing and why. Avoid getting in line. Yes, it is impressive you can soar through the air in your postures, but why are you doing them? How are the things you are repeating helping you, or are they? What is your intention in life each moment at a time?

It is inherent in my nature to not follow the crowd. From being a tow headed blonde growing up in a land of black hair, in Japan, I have always felt comfortable standing alone. I don't recommend it. Alone means alone. Learning to work with others, is part of the big game of life and what we are here to learn. You might be in someone's life for only a short amount of time. What are you going to do with that time? Leave a positive surplus of energy behind, or a deficit in the energy field? What are you leaving behind in your life's work? If we were to see your life in review would it be a positive contributing story or the opposite? This is the type of thought I encourage in your pursuit of yoga, or anything you approach in life. Close your eyes and take the first answer you get, trust it and know that the answer is your own personal Why. You may not like the answer and you may wish to argue it or rationalize it. Try it, ask yourself frequently and often, why are you there in that moment. If you cannot get an answer, you are probably not in the right place or your motivators are not what you thought.

I clearly remember annoying many teachers in the academic world as well as in Boy Scouts and I am sure my parents. In fact, I have been told many times by strangers and those that I believed were my friends, how annoying I can be. It is fine with me. I accept myself as I am, warts and all, as we should all do. I always hear my teacher's guru's words resounding in my head about how the highest spiritual practice is self-observation without judgement. So I am annoying, no use in beating myself up over it. Understanding why I am irritating to some is important. For I see my constant questioning as a seeking for answers and truth. Most all children are constantly curious and ask why all the time. The only reason we stop asking why is because we are told it is annoying. The world is a wonder to the new being. Everything is a mystery to be proven, explored or solved.

Not taking everything the world and people on it say at face value as the ultimate truth, but questioning why, leads to justice, freedom, liberty and equality. The great movements towards change in the way society, governments and people function have begun because a single person braved to ask why. Civil liberties, equal rights and freedom of expression have been won because a brave soul asked why. Why are things the way they are? Just because someone said they should be or because we have done it that way historically? That is not good enough. Refuse to walk on the straight and narrow or follow the norm. Stand up, stand out and ask why! Why am I doing this and what good is it doing?

I humbly thank you for your time and effort in reading this book and it is with deep gratitude that I say I hope I have helped you to begin the first step of understanding. Ask why frequently and often. Why is the studio right for me? Why is the teacher asking me to do this to my body? Why would the class lead me to this group of postures? Why am I here and what am I getting out of this? Why am I doing yoga?

Acknowledgments

Yogi Amrit Desai
Amrit Yoga and the Yoga Sutras
Yoga Network International, Inc. 2010

Diane Ross
Meditation for Miracles
CreateSpace 2012

John Mundahl
The Swami Kripalu Reader: Selected Works from a Yogic Master
Jul 7, 2014 |

Ram Das

Paramahansa Yogananda

Mahatma Ghandi

The Yoga Alliance

All the many teachers, authors, students and gurus that I have learned and grown through experiencing their teachings or words. Their generous giving has flavored and colored this inspired writing. I apologize for any mis-quotes or forgotten sources I may have invariably missed.

Made in the USA
San Bernardino, CA
12 September 2016